ANTI-DRUG MATTER

By

Deviled Tongue

This book is a work of fiction partly
inspired by true events and life
experiences. Names, characters, places,
and incidents either are a product of the
author's imagination or are used
fictitiously. Any resemblance to actual persons, living
or dead, events, or locales is entirely coincidental.

Library of Congress Cataloging-IN-Publication Data

ISBN:9780615782553

Printed in the United States of America

Anti-Drug Matter

Deviled~Tongue

ACKNOWLEDGEMENTS

Every author's acknowledgment, while it can be general is personal to that author. In no particular order, I am extending heartfelt thanks and gratitude: To my first grade teacher Mrs. Band, Hercules Medical Group, my brother Valentino, my sisters Valerie, Veronica and Vivian, Faythe Brannon, Majita Dalton, Yolanda Russell, Hans Burns, Jackie Koleshnick and Family, Carmelita Frazier, Nikki Robinson, Mark and Rachel Bradshaw, Harol Mata and Emmanuel Rosales, Rena DeGrella for sharing ideas, Troy Green for his friendship, Tamra Spearman-Enoch for supporting my craft and being a fan, Leticia Smalls - (my ride or die-partner in crime) who always inspired me to be ultra-creative, Amy Yeung whose word skills challenged me to rethink my thinking, my cousin Alfonso Washington for his constant encouragement and current events updates, Jerome Fortson for always checking in, my mother and Melvin for keeping me spiritually grounded, Lena Colon who always kept on the lookout for opportunities for me to have this book published, Marla Warren-the mother of my child for letting me type all night despite the higher electric bill, my daughter Nykemah for critiquing my creativity, and Anthony Ferguson for supporting my passion; rest in peace, 'Phoenix'.

Dedicated to my mother who
thought about becoming a police
officer;
and my entire family who didn't want me to become
one.

PREFACE

This isn't actually the first printing; it's the first publishing. Anti-Drug Matter was written in 2004 with the intent of being published, but agents and publishers both, rejected the manuscript. I decided that the story was too dated to put out as it was. So I kept the central theme, but reworked the characters and situations.

Thanks to technology and online DIY availability, I am now able to bring this masterpiece of my imagination to you on an electronic platform. To be fair, a fictional book is a wonderful literary voice that has no equal. Thanks to *E-books and audio books, one will still be entertained by an author's creativity; but having come from the typewriter era, nothing beats sitting down with a good book and reading it to yourself, or aloud to someone else.

*Do electronic books and audio books remove something that the writer is trying to convey? No. A good story is a good story. Marketing and Promotion of a book will always be a factor as well. Because of time and space, or a lack thereof, these mediums are a welcome format for writers and readers born before the beginning of 2005. Paperback and hardcover novels may or may not totally vanish. But how many people today have a mini library in their dwelling, consisting of various books including but not limited to: fiction, nonfiction, encyclopedias, a dictionary, DIY books, self-help books, cookbooks, children's books, and crossword puzzle or coloring books? Most people will probably have a Bible, but that ideally would be the only book still in printed form in their possession.

I started out as a songwriter, and to my credit received recognition from an ASCAP songwriting contest for my effort. I also received a favorable critique from a record pool that evaluated my first recording. Alas, neither of those wonderful organization's experiences landed me a recording contract. So I ventured out on my own, but due to lack of capital, assistance, and know-how, I ended up with a name and a product but no career.

Life happens and life gets in the way. Sometimes you get discouraged and feel like you've wasted your time and your efforts to become a professional performer. It happens overnight for some, while others just have to stay passionate and determined to become successful.

I chose the pseudonym Deviled Tongue, because controversy creates conversation. I want you to listen to me. I'm not saying I know it all, nor am I saying I am always right. I'm just one person with an opinion, but it is an opinion that most people tend to agree with. My name is the total opposite of 'evil outspoken'. Instead, I want to get your attention, and explain things to you in a unique way that will hold your attention as well as help you understand. Some people tell me I should have become a schoolteacher. But referring back to what I mentioned earlier about E- books and audiobooks, I am teaching. And it's my hope that you will learn something of value from my lessons, as well as be entertained.

The 'Deviled~Tongue' has spoken.

PROLOGUE

New York City; present day. After all that occurred in years past, one constant, remains the same: the individuals who make up law enforcers assigned to confiscate narcotics, have molded what relationships should ideally emulate; both professional and personal.

Anti-Drug Matter is a visionary Red, White, and Blue portrayal of courage, success, love, and tragedy as experienced by two twin brothers who are police detectives. Shamel is assigned to a special NYPD narcotics unit. Preacher is with the Alexandria, Va. Police Department drug enforcement team.

Mstislab, (pronounced mist-slab) a notorious rising crime lord within the Russian Mafia is planning to capitalize off the frenzy permeated by sweeping changes to the assault rifle ban and the uptick in gun violence nationwide. Mstislab already has a flourishing drug trade, but is about to up the ante in his opportunistic endeavor to become the largest crime boss on the East Coast.

Unbeknownst to the twins and crime lord, their paths (which had been indirectly intertwining), are going to cross in a violent final battle for control of the city – and possibly a Nation.

AUTHOR'S NOTE

This book is a work of fiction partly inspired by true events and life experiences. Names, characters, places, and incidents either are a product of the author's imagination or are used fictitiously. Any resemblance to actual persons, living or dead, events, or locales is entirely coincidental.

Also, it's my mind that has the real battles. ☺

Twitter@DeviledTongue

Anti~Drug Matter

Chapter One

Ash from the cigarette danced in the crisp, chilly October breeze while the butt itself bounced and rolled from Mstislab's flicking it away, as he blew the remaining smoke through his nostrils. He was obviously disgruntled, but did not express himself verbally. His body language was the clue to his displeasure; arms crossed, feet apart. His head was erect with a scowl on his face and a fixed gaze. He was not in a good mood at all.

"Slab, I see him coming now." -- his *Pakhan, and right-hand man, Seryoga announced. (*Underboss in Russian.)

'Slab' was the nickname Mstislab became known by, after his many brutal strong-arm enforcement tactics against rivals, and workers who either disobeyed him or made a mistake. Seryoga was Mstislab's sidekick from day one. Fiercely loyal, Seryoga would ensure Mstislab's orders were carried out. He even went as far as unleashing brutal punishment on his own to those who failed to comply. However, Seryoga demonstrated cowardice. He never took it upon himself to actually kill anyone. In fact, unless Mstislab committed the killing (which he did, most of the time), Seryoga delegated the task to a **Brigadier (**Soldier in Russian) within their crime family. It has been like this for a long time. Mstislab was such a hothead who was quick to pull the trigger, knife, or perform various other means of execution anyway, that he did not make an issue out of Seryoga's lack of lethal use. That issue would surface much later in their partnership, which would serve as a means to an end as well.

The headlights of the approaching vehicle seemed to weave up and down like a sine wave. Mstislab was dressed in black from head to toe. He had on a knit skull cap, three-quarter length leather jacket, scarf, denim jeans, and motorcycle boots. Mstislab was from Washington, DC. But tonight, he was conducting his business in New York – on the West Side, around 134th Street and 12th Avenue under the West Side Highway - - an area infamous for all types of shady dealings. The area had been zoned for industrial use, but plans were scrapped in New York City's budget cuts meets the fiscal requirements battle. All of the commercial owned businesses packed up and moved elsewhere. Because the area is virtually deserted, police don't bother patrolling it. Soon, the street pharmacists moved in. They were smart enough in dealing only to known clientele so they would stay low key… That was, until tonight. It was 11:40pm. The Black Hummer H2 with silver rims came to an effortless rolling stop alongside Mstislab and Seryoga. Though the dark tinted windows were up, the system which was blaring some kind of Electro-House music was audible. Mstislab bared his teeth, and motioned with a swift slice of his right hand across his neck for the music to be muted. Both the SUV and radio were turned off, and the lone driver exited.

"Hey, Mstislab, I'm s-"

"Late. Very - late." Mstislab replied, cutting off the lone driver's apology. Mstislab said it in a monotone, firm and calm voice. A nervous energy began to build.

Mstislab glared at the driver; a slender, young Russian male with acne. He was wearing a throwback jersey, jeans, sneakers, and a baseball cap with 'NY' stitched on it. The driver put up his hands in a sort of surrender...

"Mstislab, that's why I called and left a message on your cell, I told you, I ran into a problem."

"Oh, you sure as hell did! I got your message, and there's no excuse. At least not one that I'm going to accept." Mstislab replied still in calm, but more intense tone.

The driver continued, "There was a lot of traffic on I-95, probably from all that road work. Then I ran into a bad accident on the turnpike. And you know how the GW Bridge is backed up and all."

"You are screwing up my *conveyor belt*! I need to get to Boston to initiate things there. The only reason I'm even in New York right now is because Seryoga had to pick up his new LS 460. Since you were going to be tardy, I made the decision to tell you off here, rather than waste time and gas going up north. I depend on

you, to make the necessary transport on time. But thanks to **you**, my connection in 'New England' won't be available by the time we were supposed to arrive!"

"I didn't mean to mess things up, Mstislab. Seryoga called me and told me to stop here instead of going to Massachusetts. But when I asked to speak to you, he wouldn't let me!" -- the driver accusingly and crossly said to Mstislab.

"I didn't want to talk to you. Not after receiving that message! No matter how you try to shift the blame, excrement rolls downhill, and you, are at the bottom of the landing!"

"Mstislab, believe me, I – I wouldn't have come if I had known there would be so much drama!"

That comment infuriated Mstislab. He got right in the young driver's face, like a drill instructor chastising a recruit. Mstislab bellowed, "You wouldn't have come? You, wouldn't have come? Since when do you refuse orders to me? Who do you think you're talking to?"

"Mstislab, I meant I would've, but, well, like I just would've – well, when I said that, I meant I wouldn't have gotten into all that traffic!"

"I dis-tinctly heard you say 'I wouldn't have come!' No matter what you meant Yuri, this shipment is late! If you were a 'period' the belly would be showing by now!" Mstislab snarled. Seryoga whistled and looked away, smirking at the comment. The driver was nervous, and began to squirm a bit. Mstislab walked to the back of the Hummer, tapped the rear door and snapped "Open it!" to the driver, who looked as if he was ready to run away. Unlocking the trunk from the inside, the driver stood by his door, but was motioned by Mstislab to walk towards the rear of the SUV. Seryoga came and stood right next to the driver, somewhat escorting him in Mstislab's direction. Mstislab was looking in the back of the Hummer in the cargo area, and slowly shaking his head from left to right. In a heavy Russian accent, he uttered "*Бog". (*God in Russian, pronounced 'loch'.) "It's a good thing my order for that extra Ecstasy was canceled, or

I'd be the laughingstock of every dealer in the city!" Mstislab looked at the driver and flashed an evil grin, which transformed into a frown. "Why is only half of the shipment here?" The driver started backing up, but he didn't realize Seryoga was behind him. Seryoga shoved the driver forward, making him bang his head on the open rear door. The dull thud and the driver's howl of pain were in accord as the driver stumbled backwards, but regained his footing. He turned around with his back towards the Hummer, now facing Mstislab and Seryoga who both had their arms folded.

"Mstislab, please. Like I said, I was trying to call you."

"Maybe he needs the fat, black man – *de* '4Genie', eh?" Seryoga mused. Both he and Mstislab laughed heartily, as the driver began stammering with his sentences.

"I, I (gulping) – Yo, Mstislab. Check it out. I did like you said. I came out of Richmond, long after I had contact with the Pakhans' and Brigadiers' in Norfolk. I stopped in 'DC' at the safehouse. Divvied up what had to go there, and then continued on to Baltimore Plaza to do the car switch."

"And what happened?" Mstislab growled.

"Yo, check it out. Totally unexpected, a Maryland State Trooper pulled into the plaza, maybe on a routine check or whatever. Me, Jaska, and Nunchaku got nervous and rushed the exchange! In the confusion I ended up leaving half of the product with them. But you know them! They ain't gonna short change you! They know better!"

The driver was almost pleading; his tone one of fear, as Mstislab and Seryoga kept eyeing him down. If looks could kill, blood would have been flowing out of the driver's body at this very moment. Doom was imminent -- the only question was, when. Mstislab slowly rotated his head, emitting a cracking sound from his neck. Then without warning, he punched the driver in the face knocking him backwards again, into the open rear of the Hummer. Mstislab then slipped his left hand into the right side of his leather jacket.

Seryoga pulled a butterfly knife out of his pants pocket, and after flicking it open, began cleaning his nails with the blade tip.

"How in the name of Capitalism, do you know or even guarantee that they won't stiff me? You the 'Rasputin' of honest *Bratva (*Brotherhood) or something?" Mstislab questioned. "On top of it all, you were entrusted with getting the shipment and you failed! But I'll speak to your Pakhan about that!"

While nursing his bruised and swollen face, the driver responded, "Mstislab, please! It's my first time with a long distance shipment on my own!"

"And your last." Mstislab said with callousness.

"Mstislab, as far as Jaska and Nunchaku go, I know these guys! I made runs with and for them on a regular basis! I know that if they were gonna rob you, -"

"They would come up missing - just like you!" Mstislab countered. He then whipped out a Baby Eagle 9mm, pulled the slide back, and pointed it at the driver's head.

"Mstislab, No!" the driver screamed, but Mstislab wasn't having it.

Turning the weapon sideways and lowering it towards the driver's torso, Mstislab applied pressure to the trigger and fired three rounds into the driver's body. The driver crumpled to the ground, blood pouring out of his wounds.

"Search him for valuables. Phone, cash, condoms." Mstislab ordered Seryoga, as he holstered his gun. A dog could be heard barking a short distance away. Mstislab looked around wildly, trying to make sure there were no witnesses to the shooting. Seryoga pulled a pair of latex gloves out of his pocket, and after donning them began searching the driver's pockets, taking all the items he discovered. Finally, he took his Butterfly knife, and sliced off the driver's right ear lobe with a diamond studded earring in it, before leaving him to die.

"Ok, the mutilation part is really nasty; I just have to let you know." Seryoga said to Mstislab.

"Make sure you practice sterile technique. Roll it up in the glove. I want that lobe to show Jaska, Nunchaku, and everybody else what will happen to them if they screw up like good 'ol Yuri, here! Right, Yuri?" Mstislab said.

Mstislab kicked the driver in his side and spat on him. The driver's body jerked and he grunted as a spontaneous reaction to being kicked, but otherwise he lay motionless. Mstislab slammed the rear door of the Hummer closed, then walked around to the driver's side and got in. After starting it, he pressed the seek button on the satellite radio console and tuned in to a station playing classic rock music. He then glanced at the floor on the passenger side and was pleasantly surprised. Reaching over, Mstislab picked up a Glock 9mm handgun. At that moment, his face lit up, as if he had the most brilliant idea in the world. Tossing the Glock over his shoulder, it hit the edge of the rear seat and fell to the floor back on the passenger side. Seryoga, having finished his task pulled up next to Mstislab in a Black Lexus LS 460, with a temporary 20 day non-resident certificate in the back window. Mstislab had the driver's side window on the Hummer down, and was lighting up a cigarette.

"I want some pizza." he said to Seryoga.

"*Slab*, what's the plan now? You do realize we have to go back and get the rest of that shipment." Seryoga replied.

"Patience, Seryoga. I just came up with another idea, and this will solidify my position in the underworld. Yuri left a firearm in this vehicle. A lot of good it did him, eh?" Both chuckle. "I have a new endeavor that will net us millions! But first, I will need more funds."

"You could borrow from -"

"No." Mstislab interrupted, cutting Seryoga off. "We will use our own cash. Since we have to head back anyway, we'll stop off in Atlantic City. There I can sell off the rest of the Ecstasy, and collect some money owed to us for protection. I may even play a few rounds of High Limit Craps. We will be coming back to New York, and eventually head up to Boston. First,

I need to contact my military brethren. I want all of this set up by next May, when they come into town."

Seryoga looked puzzled; Mstislab continued. "It's the best way to bring in a sizeable shipment for distribution, without raising suspicion. But we'll discuss it more once I've set the meeting up."

Mstislab put the Hummer in drive, rolled a few feet, and then made a screeching U-turn. He passed Seryoga and accelerated, but Seryoga was right behind him as they headed towards the highway, leaving the smell of burning rubber, and Yuri in the darkness. The only sound that lingered in the stillness of the chilly night was Yuri's faint but audible moaning of pain. He was still breathing, but barely alive. He began shivering, then mildly convulsing as he slowly descended into hypovolemic shock. Trying to alleviate the pain, he curled up into a ball on his right side. Lying on his right forearm, he grabbed at the asphalt while clutching his stomach with his left hand. He shivered, shivered, shivered –

and slowly succumbed into the 'Grim Reaper's' custody.

Chapter Two

Shamel typed furiously, trying to keep pace with the three chat message conversations going on at once on his social network. He was chatting with his girlfriend Nova, (who was being flirtatious as usual), and two officers from Brooklyn he knew. Shamel had previously been in a chat room created by another officer online. The discussion was centered on a buy and bust occurrence in Brooklyn with a deadly end result.

"That situation dictated wearing a vest. You know now they sell body armor thin enough where it can't be detected under clothing." Shamel typed and hit 'Send' to 'SexyDvice'.

"(Chime) I know, Shamel. But we're all equally upset over the communication breakdown. His backup never heard the 10-13 radio call. I wish your unit had been there."

"(Chime) Hey! You're taking too long to reply to my replies! Who else are you chatting with?" Nova IM'd.

Instead of responding to Nova, Shamel IM'd 'SexyDvice' back.

"Detective Blake shouldn't have entered that Brownstone without his backup. He knew those perpetrators were armed."

"(Chime) But he'd won their confidence, Shamel. What he didn't know was they planned to set him up to be robbed. Once they realized he was a cop, they chose to kill him."

Shamel then IM'd 'NucrisTluv'.

"Any leads on the shooter?"

"(Chime) He's still on the run, but you know they locked down Brooklyn from the expressway to the bridges and the Belt Parkway. Checkpoints all over the place."

"(Chime) Um, Shamel? Hello! Remember me? Your soon to be ex, if you don't start paying me some attention!" 'Novxxx' (Nova's screen name) IM'd Shamel.

"Hold on, Nova. BRB (Be right back)" Shamel typed and sent to Nova.

"(Chime) HOLD ON FOR WHAT, OR SHOULD I SAY WHO?" Nova IM'd back.

Shamel ignored Nova's IM, and responded back to 'SexyDvice'.

"I don't mean to be critical. But if my unit was the one handling that undercover investigation, we would have infiltrated the gang and been selling alongside them, not still buying from them. We get arrested together, then just vanish before the indictments come in. That's how you take down a drug gang in today's wars. I haven't seen the news. Did the Commissioner and Mayor hold a press conference yet?"

"(Chime) That's taking place as we speak."

"(Chime) I bet if I was between **your** legs right now, you wouldn't be telling me to 'hold on'!" Nova IM'd Shamel. But before Shamel could IM her back, 'SexyDvice' chimed in again.

"(Chime) Shamel, call me tomorrow at the station. My husband needs to use the computer right now."

"Ok, good chatting with you, Olivia. Take care. Guess I'll see you at the service." Shamel IM'd back.

"(Chime) Yeah, unfortunately, right? Have a good one, Sha! Be safe for the sistas, and your sisters and brothers in Blue!"

"I will. Have a good one, too!"

"(Chime) Bye." - 'SexyDvice' IM'd as her final response before logging off.

"(Chime) Shamel, my computer is running slow, and I may get knocked off line again. If you send an IM and I fail to respond right away, you know why." 'NuCrisTluv' IM'd.

"(Chime) You're trifling, and I don't like you very much right now!" Nova IM'd right behind 'NuCrisTluv'.

Shamel's fingertips were sweaty. He responded to Nova's IM first...

"I said 'hold on!'"

"(Chime) Yeah, I'ma hold on all right... hold on to cursing you out! You know I don't like being ignored!" Nova responded.

Shamel clicked on 'NucrisTluv's' chat and typed, "Sorry, Nichelle, I got caught up." He clicked 'send' and waited about 30 seconds for a response, but didn't receive one. Shamel typed another message…"Nichelle, you still there?" and clicked 'send'. This time, a window message popped up reading 'Chat session has ended.' "She got knocked off-line. Oh well." Shamel thought out loud. He turned his attention back to Nova, seeing that she was still logged on. "Ok, baby, I'm all yours." Shamel IM'd to Nova. He waited a full minute, but after no response, IM'd her again. "Come on, Nova! Don't be mad. Please?" Another minute passed, and Nova still didn't respond. Just as Shamel was about to send her a third IM, she finally replied.

"(Chime) Oh, now of a sudden I matter. Well, you're gonna wait for **me** now, until I'm ready to talk to you again!"

"Are you ready now? How about now? Maybe now?" Shamel teased in his reply.

"(Chime) You're lucky I do like you, sometimes anyway! Log off and call me. Been looking forward to a human **convo** with you!"

"Speak to you verbally in a bit! Love you!"

"(Chime) Love you more!"

Shamel logged off and shut down his computer. As soon as he did, Nova called on his cell phone.

"Hey!" Shamel answered. "Thought you wanted me to call you..."

"Hey..." a soothing, sultry voice responded. "Why can't you focus on me more often?"

"I focus on you every day."

"You must have me confused as one of your *C.I.'s (*Confidential Informant), 'cause I sure don't get the attention **I** deserve!"

"Nova, stop. If I don't pay you as much mind as you say, how do I always manage to come to your rescue when you need it most?"

"You're supposed to come to my rescue when I call you! I'm going to see if they have a 'Girlfriends' for Dummies' book, and make sure I autograph it just for you!"

"Oh, you think you're funny. Almost as funny as the time you tried paying for groceries with a 'Metrocard'!"

"I was tired and not **paying** attention! Besides, just like with cell phone *apps*, that process could become a reality one day."

"Maybe. But until then, as far as the deli is concerned, you earned the 'Real Drop-outs from **CUNY (**City University of New York)' award!"

"Uh-uh! No you didn't! You, you… hahahahhah!"

Nova could not contain her laughter, and neither could Shamel at that point. They always kidded like this. Shamel loved Nova, and Nova worshipped the ground Shamel walked on. They met three years ago at the Public Library, and have held a steady relationship ever since. Their conversation lasted about forty minutes. Nova playfully scolded Shamel for not being fast enough with his IM's to her; Shamel retorted by daring her to find someone better than him. They talked about the shooting in Brooklyn. They talked about taking a cruise to the Caribbean or

Cancun. They talked about living together, which was the beginning to the end of their chat.

"Sure you're ready for me to be in your presence almost 24 hours a day?" Nova asked.

"Unless *you done* cut a deal with your landlord on the side, I won't mind sharing space with you! Thought you said your roommates were annoying anyway." Shamel replied.

"There's four of us in a three bedroom loft. That's how I get away with paying only $300 a month. I have my own room as you know. But the 'Goth' chicks and the herbal, holistic, Hindu 'hippo' make living here a reality show with no camera crew!" Nova jeered.

"I'm not that easy to get along with. But that's the beauty of a two bedroom apartment. You get on my nerves, and I kick you out to the other room." Shamel answered.

"I always knew you had a motive for that two bedroom. Thought you had some other 'B' up in there you was hiding out."

"Nah, you the only 'B' for me."

"Watch your mouth, or you won't be with this '<u>B</u>', Shamel!"

"Good thing is, you won't have to worry about the rent with me. I'll take care of us."

"That's so sweet of you! Me with these lame temp positions. Days here, evenings there… (Sigh), I've got to find something permanent, Shamel."

"You will! Gotta stay positive and encouraged for that income to come in!"

"Yeah, but try telling that to <u>my creditors!</u> Maybe I should join the police force. Then **I** can tell the School Safety Division to start assigning more cops to truancy duty. Every time I look around, all I see are kids acting a fool and causing mayhem when they should be in school."

"Kinda hard for them to be in school when they can't fit into the classroom."

"You're no help! Why don't you be proactive and use your lights and siren to trap and drag them to class?"

"Because I only use my lights and siren when I'm gonna be late for roll call."

"Hmmm, Roll Call. Is that when the Pillsbury Doughboy notifies **you**? (Imitating giggle of Pillsbury Doughboy)."

"Wha – oh no you didn't!"

"Come on, Sha, this is me you're talking to! Your significant other. Better half. (And in a low whisper) Wifey?"

"Huh, what did you say? I think I need you to repeat yourself, cause it sounded like you said 'spicy'!" Shamel teased.

Nova took a deep breath, then spoke slowly and loudly. "I said, W-I-F – (beep)" - She was interrupted by her 'Call Waiting' notification. "Ok, now who is this? Caller unknown."

"Don't answer it then." Shamel urged.

"It could be a job, Sha."

"This late?"

"(Beep) - Hey, I keep my windows of opportunity wide open."

"That's why you have *bats*!"

"Ha-ha, you're about as (beep) hilarious as a dentist with no teeth! Hold on."

"Holding." - Shamel replied.

Nova clicked over to the other call. As Shamel patiently waited, he gazed at a photo of Nova and himself, taken at a mall photo booth. His thoughts immediately took him back to when they first met...

It was a nice, warm early Saturday afternoon. Shamel was off duty, and decided he would head to the New York Public Library just to get out of the apartment. Deciding to check his email, he scoped the room thinking he would have to wait for a computer when he noticed one was available. Shamel hurried over to it, only to bump into a woman who was trying to gain access to the same computer as well.

"Excuse me." Shamel said.

"Excuse me!" the woman replied politely, but in a flustered tone of voice.

"I believe I was here first." Shamel said.

"I didn't see you waiting around. As soon as I walked in, I saw this one was free!"

"Look, miss. I'm not here to argue. I just want to check my email, then be on my way."

"Well, you'll have to check your email after I check mine!" the woman snapped, edging her way onto the computer. Shamel was about to protest when she said to him, "Look, honestly I won't be long. My phone died and it was a message about a job. Why don't you just wait next to me, and I'll let you have it right after I check. Promise."

Shamel grumbled, but complied with the request. The woman signed on, gave the mouse a few quick clicks, then let out a dejected sigh.

"Position filled. And they call me just to tell me that." she said to herself, but audible enough where Shamel heard her. "I'm done. See how fast that was? Thank you, sir."

"Uh, looking for a job?" Shamel said to her somewhat awkwardly.

"Been looking. All I get is the usual. Position filled, job no longer available, or no response at all. But thanks anyway." the woman replied, as she signed out of her email account and began walking away.

"Um, hold on. Maybe you should, well, I guess what I'm trying to ask is, how many sites is your resume posted on?"

"It doesn't matter."- She sighed again in exasperation. "Besides, I thought you were eager to check your own email."

"Hey, it's only email. Probably spam at that. I'm not in a rush, if you want to keep looking."

The woman stopped and looked at Shamel.

"Is this supposed to be an offer I can't refuse?" she said in a soft, seductive tone.

"Well, either one of us could have waited for another computer. But, I kinda liked waiting for the one you were using."

"And why is that?" she graciously challenged.

"The scent you left behind. 'Forever Red'. One of my favorite colors."

A radiant smile formed across the woman's face. She walked back up to the computer and signed on again.

"A man who knows perfumes. I admire that. I had a little job selling samples before I quit. The owner was stiffing everybody out of their pay with that salary plus commission scheme. Before that, I was a medical biller in a private doctor's office. Then, unbeknownst to me, someone found out he was committing Medicaid fraud. He was shut down, and I've been looking for work ever since. Speaking of perfume samples, I like the scent of your cologne. It smells so spring-like!"

"It's 'Downey'. I do my laundry, then shower and dress."

"Oops. What do I know? I can barely afford dryer sheets!"

"Hey, I understand. You're on a budget. But if we get to know each other better, I'll have your clothes smelling 'April fresh' too!"

"Maybe I don't want you washing my panties."

"I have to get them off you first, heh-heh!"- Shamel snickered.

"Damn, you bold! But, that's ok. I could use a masculine influence in my life. That is, if you're **really** single; no baby momma, no down-low lovers, no side chick jump off."

"I feel you, and yes I am **really** single! How about you? No jealous boyfriend trying to reach you on your dead cell phone right now?"

"Ok, that's not funny, and just like we don't want no broke brothas, guys don't want no broke 'sisters'."

"Then what makes me the exception?"

"I never said I was broke, I just said I'm unemployed. Watch 'Mad Money' on CNN if you need a breakdown. But seriously, just haven't found a guy I like who likes me who has likes that I like. Then, like I meet you. Maybe we can like each other – on 'Facebook' even."

"Gonna need an email address."

"I'm aware of that. Since I'm checking mine, tell me yours, and I'll email you."

"Why not just tell me?"

"Who writes phone numbers and addresses down anymore? This will also ensure, and insure that you don't misplace my information. That is unless, again, you're not **really** single." - The woman stated with a firm emphasis.

"Really? **Really?"** Shamel mocked. "I am single, unless..." (He paused for a moment, which caused the woman to raise her eyebrows in anticipation of a confession.) "You consider my twin brother."

"You're a twin? That's so cool! Now you and he aren't gonna play that 'bull' where you date me one night, and he dates me the next, are you?" she questioned.

"(Laughing) He doesn't even live in this state! But we can always talk about that other part of my life in the present future."

"Well, sending this email would secure that, if I knew your name and email address."

"Of course! It's Shamel, spelled like it sounds. My email address is long.
It's 'Twincarcerated@ugotmail.cyberPostOffice'."

"I like that!" the woman replied, as she typed her information in the email. "Well, thanks Shamel. It was nice meeting you, and I appreciate you letting me use the computer first. Course you wouldn't have gotten my identity if you hadn't (giggle)."

"So, then I'll see you again?" Shamel asked cautiously.

"Damn, he's good looking and intelligent!" the woman cynically replied to Shamel, as she walked away for the last time.

"Hey, I thought you were gonna surf for jobs!" Shamel yelled after her.

"No, I have to be going. Got another job interview later this afternoon. You believe that, on a Saturday? My life. But check your email, **now**. That is, if you **really** want to see me again! Take care!"

The woman walked away. Shamel signed on, and went to his email account. He didn't see any new or unknown emails right away, so he clicked on his junk email folder, and there it was; 'KitnKaboodle79': 'Just met U in the Library'. Shamel clicked on the email, and was delighted with the contents…

"Name: Novaline (Nova for short – like Super Nova!), Age: You'll learn that if we get past this email. Birthday: November 12. Stats: Belief in God. Love long drives, walks, talks. Have own car. No job right now – but you knew that. Roommates, no animals, no kid(s), and no man - yet; Position open. Non-smoker, drink if offered one. Cell: 347-555-3210. Any additional info including but not limited to, address, favorite color, education level, etc. is up to you!-☺"

At that moment, Nova clicked back over to Shamel.

"Shamel,"

"Still here, 'babycakes'"

"Let me take this call. It's my friend Yuki, the one who just gave birth."

"Ha! You don't need to be talking to her!"

"You ain't right! Men just don't get it!"

"No, but we sure like to give it!"

"Creep! On that note, I'll speak to you later. Gonna be up? Are you going to be home? It's not like you have some place to be now."

"Yeah, I ain't going nowhere."

"Ok, cause you know what I'll do if I call and-"

"Yea-yea-yea-yea-yea-yea-yea-yea-yea-yea-yea-yea-yeah!" Shamel butted in. "Go and give your 'girl' some P.F.A."

"Some what?" - Nova exclaimed.

"Psychological First Aid!" Shamel replied, laughing.

"Oh! Thought it was something sexual. Never know with *yo* ass! Love you, Sha."

"I love you more." Shamel replied

"I love you, more." Nova replied back.

"You ain't lied yet! Bye."

"Bye-bye." Nova replied softly, before both of them ended their call.

Chapter Three

The timing was perfect. No sooner had Shamel hung up from Nova, a text message came in. It was his friend Tino, a police officer from *Manhattan Boro 35th*. The message read, "Got a body out here on 12th Av off 125th Street. Eyewitness. Could be for you, so get here asap!" Shamel texted back, "I'm on it. Thx." Shamel placed his phone inside his pants pocket, and got ready to leave. From time to time, Tino would call Shamel whenever he thought a potential drug case was evident. Shamel of course appreciated the 'heads-up' as well. Now he frowned in concentration. He went to the closet, pulled out his gun case and took an ankle holster from a rack. He opened the case and took out his treasured backup weapon; a Ruger .357 snub-nose Magnum. Flicking open the cylinder, Shamel then took out a 5 shot speed reloader, and chambered each round in one motion. After securing the Magnum in the holster, Shamel fastened it to his right inner ankle. He went into his bedroom and grabbed his wallet, keys, and gold detective shield off the dresser. Now out in the living room, Shamel headed to the hallway closet and grabbed his full length leather trench coat. He put on his coat, pulled a wool knit hat out of the trench pocket, and placed his shield around his neck. He resembled a thug more than a cop, but being an undercover officer affiliated with the unit he was assigned to, his manner of dress assured that he could play a more effective role of blending in. Shamel had an NFL player physique. At 6'1" and 260lbs, he looked menacing – especially when his facial expression made *the look*. People said he looked mean; like he was going to kill them - then keep on killing them even after they were dead. Shamel was used to comments such as, "If you could only see that look on your face right now." He couldn't, so he just took everybody's word for it and made it work for him. Being a twin, Shamel's brother could produce *the look* as well. But his brother was more laid back. It was just a trait people who knew the twins took notice of.

Shamel began to make his way out the door when he stopped short… "Damn!" he exclaimed out loud, slapping his forehead. He turned around, took off his coat, and shield. Upon opening the hall closet this time, Shamel took out his windbreaker, and a bullet-proof vest. The vest was a birthday gift from his brother. By coincidence, Shamel had purchased the exact same style of vest to give to him. So, in a moment that was captured on video, the brothers' exchanged vests with each other at their birthday party, and called it 'twin-tuition'! The protective apron was a top of the line 'DuPont' Kevlar body armor vest -- the kind that would even stop Teflon coated 'cop killer' bullets! Shamel donned the vest, put on the windbreaker, his trench again and his shield. He placed it under the zipper of the windbreaker so that it was not visible. Finally, he adjusted the hood of the windbreaker so it fell outside the collar of his trench, then he looked in the mirror. The extra apparel made him appear huskier than usual, but he knew it was a necessary precaution. Shamel prepared to exit the apartment once again when he stopped and looked up at the ceiling. In a solemn yet symbolic gesture, Shamel said out loud,

"Watch my back, Detective Blake. You too, dad." Shamel then took his right hand and drew a cross with his index and middle fingers from his forehead to the middle of his chest, and across from shoulder to shoulder like he had observed Catholics do. Though Shamel was not Catholic, he admired that particular show of spirituality, and adopted it for himself.

Shamel left the apartment and proceeded outside. He walked over to his car, and caught an attitude when he saw what appeared to be a ticket on his windshield. On closer examination, he discovered it was an orange flyer designed to resemble a New YorkCity parking summons envelope. Shamel pulled it from under the windshield wiper blade and quickly viewed it. Partially in bold lettering, it read; "**This** could have been **Another Parking Ticket!** Now fines are as high as **$115! $265** for Tractor-trailers! Why take chances with **your BENJAMINS', LINCOLNS', OR YOUR JEFFERSONS'?** Save, with the first in War against parking, first in Peace of mind, and first in

AFFORDABLE RATES! WASHINGTON's Park-A-Lot! Reasonable rates! No Lie..."

Shamel didn't even bother reading the rest. He crumpled up the flyer and swatted it down the street. "Help keep 'Sanitation' employed!" he thought to himself. Pressing the remote on his keys, Shamel deactivated his car alarm and got in. After adjusting the rear view mirror, he took his NYPD Vehicle Identification placard from the sun visor and placed it on the dash. He never left it displayed in the window as a precaution from vandals, thieves, and to keep his police occupation anonymous. Shamel's block was pretty decent though, compared to the surrounding area. His apt building was one of the new Housing Preservation and Development initiatives, with rent based on income. His apartmentt had space too! Most of the residents in this working class black neighborhood kept to themselves, including Shamel. He didn't think he was better than or too good to socialize with his neighbors, but emulating a quiet existence helped him maintain a low profile. His neighbors didn't know who he was or what he did for a living, and he wanted to keep it that way.

Shamel started his Acura ILX and pulled off the block. Once he was around the corner on 'Malcolm X Boulevard', he put his red beacon on the dash and activated his flashers. (As a special authorized law enforcer, he was allowed to outfit his personal vehicle with emergency equipment.) Shamel figured he'd use the siren intermittently rather than have it blaring all the way down the street. Two quick 'yelps', and the few cars that were in front of him pulled to the right. He now had a clear left lane of traffic. Shamel deduced that the quickest way to the West Side Highway would be to take 140th Street Westbound to Riverside Drive, then Riverside all the way to 125th Street. Turning onto 140th Street, Shamel got behind a black livery car that seemed to be refusing to yield. Shamel hit the 'phaser' and air horn effects of his siren, and watched the cab nearly sideswipe parked cars on both sides of the street as it veered left, then abruptly to the right to get out of Shamel's way. Shamel lowered his passenger window and pulled alongside the cab. The driver, a middle aged male who appeared to be of African ethnicity looked nervous. Shamel was about to say something, but gave the cab driver *the look* instead, and drove on. "Probably cursing me out in 'Swahili' right now!" - Shamel chuckled to himself. He drove another few city blocks until he reached his destination. Shamel arrived just in time to see the FDNY ambulance slowing departing. Its emergency lights and siren were off, and the crew seemed in no hurry to be going anywhere. Shamel also noticed the four police cars from the 35th precinct still at the scene, three with their emergency lights flashing. The four vehicles formed a semi-circle around the driver's corpse, which was covered with a sheet. Yellow crime scene tape was tied to lamp and sign posts from one side of the street to the other, forming a square around the police. Shamel stopped and parked. He pulled his shield out from his windbreaker, then got out the Acura and closed the door, leaving it slightly ajar. He headed directly towards Officer Tino Valentine-Brown – his friend, and the one who texted him about the incident. Shamel acknowledged the other seven officers, and then spoke to Tino.

"Nice night for mayhem. Not even Halloween yet." - Shamel said to Tino, while they engaged in the Afro-American cultural handshake and hug combo.

"Glad you got here before Homicide. Chances are they're gonna turn this over to you anyway, unless it gets kicked over to Major Case." Tino suggested. "911 citywide emergency dispatched the call as a carjacking with shots fired. My partner and I arrived on scene first, and found the deceased who according to the witness was alive at the time of the call."

"Um-hm!" Shamel replied, listening intently. Tino continued,

"That guy over there," Shamel turned his head and looked as Tino pointed towards a man with a dog standing off to the side. "He's the one who witnessed the crime, and tried to help the victim in his final moments. EMS pronounced him. We informed them we had to wait for Homicide, *CSU (*Crime Scene

Unit), and **OCME (**Office of Chief Medical Examiner)."

"Did the witness make the 911 call?"

"Yes. Claims he watched the whole incident from start to finish while out walking his dog. Think he'll get a medal?"- Tino cracked. He and Shamel both laughed as they approached the witness. The witness was a middle-aged Hispanic male. With him was a pure bred female Pit Bull on a leash, which began to growl and took an attack stance as Tino and Shamel approached.

"Whoa!" Shamel exclaimed, throwing up both hands, while Tino stopped short and placed his hand on his gun.

"***'Esperanza'! (***Hope) ****Sentarse! (****Sit down)" the witness commanded to the canine in a Spanish accent. "It's ok, officers. She's very well trained and not usually like this." he reassured, while pushing the Pit Bull's hind part to the ground with one hand. He offered the strap portion of the leash to the Pit Bull, which willingly took it into its mouth, then fully laid down and rolled onto its back, as the man began gently stroking her. Shamel and Tino continued to approach, until they were within adequate talk range of the witness. The witness continued to stroke the Pit Bull's stomach, as he gave Shamel an inquisitive look.

"She's in doggie heaven now, isn't she?" Shamel kidded, as Tino relaxed and nodded his head in agreement. "Good evening sir. I'm Detective Haynes, NYPD.

You've already met Officer Valentine-Brown. Would you mind explaining to me what you saw occur here tonight?"

"Not at all. I have to apologize for my dog, 'Esperanza' again. She's really very friendly. I guess being so close to that gunfire really scared her!" the witness replied with an uneasy laugh.

Shamel was uncertain at this point if this was a case he and his unit should be pursuing. His primary scene survey failed to point to anything drug related, and from what Tino relayed to him, it could have been nothing more than a fatal robbery. He knew however that any information was better than none at all. Shamel extended his right hand. To his satisfaction, the witness began to relax and open up as they shook hands.

"My name is Hector Sarmiento. I usually walk 'Esperanza' around nine or so. Tonight I got home from work late, which is why I'm out now. But anyway, I'm walking her, and she had to stop to make *caca,* which is-"

"I'm aware of what it is sir, please continue." Shamel politely interrupted.

"Well, she's just about done with her business when I hear three shots – Pop! Pop! Pop! They scared 'Esperanza' so much I couldn't calm her down at first. I was scared too! I didn't want to move until I was sure whoever was shooting was gone."

"Did you manage to get a look at the shooter?"

"No, detective. I do know there were two people though."

"You witnessed two people taking off in a car?"

"No, I saw two cars take off. I ran over to the guy they shot. He muttered that his boss shot him, and took his truck. I told 911 that someone had been shot and their vehicle was stolen. But this guy lying on the ground took his last breath once I hung up."

"Ok, sir. If you don't mind, I'm sure the Homicide division would like to take a statement from you. I appreciate your time and involvement." Shamel said.

"No problem, Detective... um, your name again?"

"Haynes." Shamel replied, extending his hand again to shake.

Tino turned to Shamel and quietly said, "What *boss* would kill you and take your vehicle?"

"Maybe the guy worked for 'Hertz on Demand'! I don't know. But anytime someone uses the term 'boss', it does sound like it's either gang and, or drug related."

"That's why I contacted you. Wanna see the body? It's not appropriately dressed for the season. Looks like whoever shot him also took a slice of his ear." Tino stated.

Shamel made a face and walked over to the covered body of the driver. He gingerly lifted up the sheet and surveyed the corpse. He looked at the face, sizing it up for recognition. Shamel then took out his phone, and took a photo of the driver's face, before letting the sheet drop back down.

"Weird." Shamel said to Tino. "I'll run his face through our database and see if any hits turn up. Maybe this isn't what it appears like. Maybe this poor guy was having an affair with his boss's wife. Kill him, take the truck she bought him, throw it in her face, get divorced, and leave her all alone while he continues banging his own mistress."

"Gee, you got it all figured out already, huh 'Shaft' – I mean, Shamel?" Tino mused.

"Keep it up; you'll be studying for that Sergeant exam on your own!" Shamel jokingly retorted.

"Hey Tino, Homicide just pulled up." Tino's partner yelled over to him.

"That's my cue to go. Thanks, Tino. I'll let you know if anything comes out of this." Shamel said.

"Always willing to look out. Have a good night." Tino replied, as they gave each other the cultural handshake/hug combo one last time before Shamel departed. He knew it was better not to intervene in what was rightfully Homicide's jurisdiction unless and until a thorough investigation dictated otherwise. He didn't have problems or rivalry with them, but he didn't want to cause any friction either by them seeing him there.

Shamel got into his car, and decided to grab a bite to eat. It was 12:36am. Heading up 125th Street, he approached the 'Apollo Theater', which had some concert activity going on. What caught his eye was the tour bus in front. Not that Shamel was into rubbernecking, but he was curious to see who the performer was, as the name was not displayed on the electronic marquee. He turned on his flashers, and stopped in the middle of the street for a brief moment. He was able to catch a glimpse of recording artist 'Felan-Tropea' who was signing autographs as she was making her way to the bus. Shamel gave a quick 'yelp' of approval from his siren, then turned off his flashers and continued on his way. Making a right turn on Adam Clayton Powell Boulevard, Shamel parked behind a silver Cadillac Escalade-EXT. He got out and entered 'White Castle' which wasn't crowded, with only four customers inside who were standing near the entrance. As soon as Shamel opened the door, a cloud of marijuana smoke hit his face. The four male patrons inside were loud and unruly, waiting for an order they placed. They were sharing a 'blunt', and all quickly glanced at Shamel with one of them even giving him *the nod,* before reengaging in their little assembly. Shamel muttered "S'cuse me." in a low but audible and firm tone of voice as he made his way to the counter. The four males were also being obnoxious, ridiculing the counterpersons…

"Damn, they taking long. This is why you don't smoke before you eat. I'm bout to jump over the counter and put 'shawty' on some bread!" one of the males commented.

"Naw, big girl in the back? She got enough meat to supply the 'Hurricane Sandy' relief effort! Hell, 'Katrina' too!" - Another male threw in.

"Son, stop babysitting that blunt, or you buying the next bag!" - A third male commented.

"Yo, miss! Don't forget my marinara sauce for those cheese sticks! Every time I come up in here and order, ya don't get it right!" the last male directed towards the servers.

"That's because they too busy being stank! Like the smell of this place ain't enough!" the second male taunted.

The all-female crew was visibly annoyed, but they continued to work in silence. One came to the window and said to Shamel "I'll be with you in a moment, sir." Shamel acknowledged her with a smile. He then pulled the windbreaker hood over his head, and leaned against the wall. He was avoiding visual contact with the rude customers, who were annoying him as well. Times like this, Shamel wished he could pull out his gun and shield, and pull rank. He knew of course he had to let things be. The four males kept heckling the counterpersons' right up until they got their food. They left, but not without hurling some final insults…

"You girls need to focus more on customer service. I better not find no nail from the salon up in my food!" the first male complained.

"If you do, just come back here, rip that 'A' off the window, and use it like toilet paper! There ain't none in the bathroom anyway!" the last male remarked, before all four walked out, laughing hysterically. Shamel watched them get into the Escalade parked out front and pull off. He turned his attention back to the counter, where all of the workers seemed relieved that the riffraff had finally gone.

"Thank you for waiting. May I have your order," the same counterperson asked Shamel.

"Yes. I'd like four fish with cheese, and a Cherry Coke." Shame replied.

"Any fries with that?"

"No, miss."

She told Shamel the total as she rang it up, then said, "Your order will be ready shortly."

"Thank you." Shamel replied with a smile.

Soon Shamel picked up his order, He thanked the counterperson again, then headed out to his car to return home. Just before he could go, his cell phone rang. Shamel opened the door of the Acura and placed his food on the seat, then retrieved his phone which had stopped ringing. Looking at the missed call log, he chuckled nervously. It was Nova.

"Oh, well. I'll just tell her she took too long to call me back and I fell asleep." Shamel thought to himself. True; he had been to a crime scene, stopped for food, and had to be at work in the morning. But he knew she didn't want to hear that! Especially since he told her he wasn't going anywhere in the first place.

Chapter Four

Shamel was preparing to enter dreamland. He double checked the alarm setting with his favorite ring tone on his cell, then knelt at his bedside and said a prayer. It was 1:49am, and he had to be at work by 7am. Though he'd already brushed his teeth, he took a final sip of his soda, then climbed into bed. Shamel turned off the lamp and lay on his side. As darkness and quiet began to meld, the nightly intruder swiftly moved in. The intruder began to pummel Shamel's eyelids, yet Shamel didn't fight back. Instead, he graciously gave up consciousness. *The Sandman* hailed his victory, and rewarded his opponent as he did every night with a free subconscious reel of visions. Tonight must have been fright night in the cerebrum however. Shamel was taken back to a rather unpleasant time – A time in his childhood. He was taken back, back…

"Dammit! You two knuckleheads better stop running through this apartment before you break something!" thundered their mother.

"But, mommy, it's raining outside!" pleaded Preacher.

"I don't give a damn if it's the second coming of Jesus! Quit running in this apartment!"

At that instant, just as if it were scripted, the phone rang – and the clatter of pots hitting the kitchen floor rang out.

"What was that? SHAMEL! If you knocked over my Black-eyed peas and Collard Greens -- PREACHER! Get the damn phone! And where is your baby sister?" their mother yelled.

"In the playpen where you left her, mom." Preacher answered.

"I should have left you **and** your brother in the playpen! Then this *fool* gets me pregnant with another one of you!"

"You mean daddy?"- Shamel who was now in his mother's presence asked innocently.

"No, I mean 'Mayor Dinkins'… Of course I mean your father!" their mother replied, annoyed.

"And didn't I tell you, Preacher to get the phone? Why is it still ringing off the hook?"

Georgia Haynes fussed at her children, as all mothers tend to do. It was Sunday afternoon. Usually after church service, the twins would go outside to play - conditions permitting of course. Sometimes their mother would accompany them with their baby sister, Venice. But the Haynes didn't attend church today. Georgia was tired, and the weather was inclement, so Shamel and Preacher horsed around indoors. But they were getting on Georgia's nerves, and about to be discharged to the area playground.

Georgia had managed to get the phone on her own, and was talking to her friend.

"Tiana, I don't want you going out of your way to pick us up. You know 'East New York' is a trek for you..."

"Stop squirting me with water!" Preacher yelled at Shamel.

"You squirted me first!" Shamel yelled back. Then Venice started crying in her playpen. Georgia had as much as she could take…

"Excuse me, Tiana. Hold on just a moment. – Preacher and Shamel, get out here NOW!"

The twins came running into the living room where Georgia was on the phone. Both of them had water spots on their shirts. Georgia gave them a stern look and said, "I'm not even going to question who's at fault. I am on the phone. The only one who should be making any kind of noise right now is your baby sister, and I will tend to her in a moment. So, before I take a belt and beat you both into foster care, I want you to go outside and play."

"Mommy…" Shamel began.

"Shut up! Don't you hear me talking to you?" Georgia interrupted. "The rain is letting up, so get outside and get some air into your lungs. Get your jackets, put on your sneakers and go."

"Mom…" Preacher started, but Georgia cut him off too.

"I am going to say the same thing I told your brother. Before I hang up this phone, you need to get outside. Because if you make me hang up, I will end up wearing the both of you out! Your father's belt is well within reach, along with the extension cord. And you know I know how to whip without causing welts. I'm not sparing the rod for either one of you. Now go!"

Preacher and Shamel went to get their outerwear, as Georgia returned to her phone conversation.

"I'm sorry, Tiana, had to chastise the boys again... They're doing fine. Just making a whole lot of noise for no good reason..."

As Preacher and Shamel were exiting the apartment, they both yelled out "Bye!" to their mother, who yelled back, "And stay off the roof!"

"We will." the boys replied lackadaisically. But once outside, Preacher and Shamel resumed their roughhousing.

The rain did let up, and now more children were coming outside, undoubtedly thrown out by their parents as well. It was early, so most of the kids played for hours as did Preacher and Shamel. They were in a community playground at the 'Louis H. Pink' Housing projects. Eventually, the number of children outside dwindled as it started getting late. Preacher and Shamel hung out until the last child they were playing with made his way home. That's when the brothers decided it was time to go in themselves. As Preacher and Shamel walked back to their building, they still engaged in roughhousing…

"Quit it, Preacher! Stop hitting me!" Shamel griped.

"See? You can't even take a little punch! You, putty!" Preacher replied, hitting Shamel on his arm again...

"I swear, Preacher, if you don't stop hitting me…"

"Ooh! Mom told you about swearing!"

"No, she said don't use the Lord's name in vain! But if you don't quit it, I'm gonna blow your chest up!"

"Yeah, right! You ain't that brave!"

Upon that, Shamel and Preacher squared off. They both put up their fists, and scowled at each other for about ten seconds. Finally, Shamel dropped his fists, then Preacher dropped his. Looking at Shamel, he chuckled. That's when Shamel threw a punch, landing it right in the center of Preacher's chest! It wasn't a hard punch, but it was enough to knock him off balance and take the wind out of him. Shamel then took off running. Preacher regained his balance and chased after Shamel. Shamel kept looking back over his shoulder to see how far away Preacher was from him. Unfortunately, it was because Shamel wasn't looking where he was going that he and Preacher ran into trouble. As Shamel rounded the corner of a building still looking behind him, he bumped into an older teenage boy. The collision nearly knocked the older boy down, but sent Shamel stumbling as well. They both regained their footing simultaneously, just as Preacher came around the corner. What happened next is everyone living in the projects' nightmare...

"Sorry, mister. I didn't see you!" gasped Shamel.

"Little idiot! You nearly knocked me down! And you got my sneakers dirty!" the older teen boy exclaimed.

"I said I was sorry!"

"*Me don* wanna here it! You need to get down on your knees, and clean off *me* sneakers!"

"Hold it, Shamel," – Preacher interjected. "Mister, he said he was sorry. Making him clean your 'kicks' is going too far!"

"You *wan* clean 'em then? '*Cause* I'm telling you, before I go home and have my dinner, somebody *gon* clean!"

"Preacher, we gotta get home. Let me just do it." Shamel pleaded.

"No! His sneakers aren't even that dirty!" Preacher countered.

"You *don* see that scuff mark? I just got these off 'Delancey Street' brand new, and here you go messing 'em up! Clean off the dirt, or else!" the teen thundered.

"Or else what?" Shamel nervously inquired.

"Ya twins? Well ya bout to get a lesson in subtraction!"

With that comment, the older teen boy reached around his back, pulled a gun out of his waistband and pointed it right at Shamel's head. Preacher jumped back startled. Shamel was petrified right where he stood. The older teen boy then pointed the gun at Preacher, but trained it right back on Shamel. Shamel was so frightened by this moment; he let his bladder go…

"Haha! Got you so scared, you *don* peed yourself!" the older boy taunted. "I should *cap* both of you! Send you to 'Kings County Hospital' in body bags! You live around here? You from the 'Pinks'? 'Cause I'll look for you every day! I'll go up in your *crib*, bust out your *moms'*, then bust a *cap* in her! Think I'm joking?"

The teen boy pressed the barrel of the gun right against Shamel's forehead.

Shamel closed his eyes. Though Preacher initially jumped back, he stepped forward and put his arm around Shamel. Shamel, still with his eyes closed, put his arm around Preacher. It definitely looked as if they were going to lose their lives together. They needed a miracle right now. That miracle came in the form of the older teen's friend who walked up…

"Man, leave those kids alone!" the other teen commanded his friend with the gun.

"Huh?" the teen with the gun replied, turning towards his friend, with a bewildered look on his face.

"Put that away before the cops see you! And you know we still got these *dime* bags on us!" his friend implored. The older teen boy actually began to comply, when his friend said to Preacher, "Wanna buy some weed? How much money you got?"

Preacher and Shamel both answered, "We don't have any."

But on that, the older teen boy re-aimed his gun at Shamel. - "Buy some weed or I'll shoot!"

The older teen's friend stepped in again; "Hey, man, don't kill no kids! You ain't got enough money to run back to the islands!" That rationale seemed to work, as the older teen boy finally put the gun away behind his back.

"Oh yeah! I was *trippin*."

Preacher looked towards the sky and silently mouthed "Thank you!" as he and Shamel let their arms drop to their sides. Shamel opened his eyes and a single tear ran down his cheek. The brothers stood fast and tried to remain stoic, hoping the betrayal of their immediate emotions would prevent the teen boys from further taunting them. But the teen who pulled out the gun decided to get some final verbal licks in…

"You two *l'il* punks are lucky my boy here ain't in no *murda* mood! Cause *me wudda* shot ya, then talked about it over breakfast in the *moning*. So consider *dis* a warning! Next time I see you, I'm adding bodies to 'Cypress Hills' cemetery!"

"Man, will you leave them kids alone and come on, already!" the other teen tried persuading.

"He *shouldn'tv* ran into me!"

"You ran into him!"

"No, I didn't!"

"Yeah, you probably did. Maybe if you didn't smoke so much *ganja,* your coordination wouldn't be off!"

"When you start taking sides for these ghetto 'street pigeons'?"

Both teens brushed past the twins without paying them any more mind. They paused for a moment which scared the twins again. But instead of the first older teen pulling out the gun, he pulled out a pack of cigarettes. After dispersing one from the pack, he lit it, returned the pack to his back pocket, and they walked on. Preacher and Shamel stood in the same spot, relieved the drama was over. But Preacher wanted payback. He decided this was a perfect opportunity to launch a sneak attack. He whispered his idea to Shamel, who protested at first. But after Preacher gave him a quick persuasive facial expression, he went along with the plan. The twins turned around and walked backwards as quickly as they could without falling. They wanted to make sure they had a good sprint distance on the two teens, but also ensure that the teens were within earshot of what they were going to yell. After the twins assessed they had a safe gap, they looked at each other, and on Preacher's mark, sounded off in unison as loud as they could…

"Ready?" Preacher asked Shamel.

"Yeah..."

"Ok. One- Two- Three! YOU CRISPY BLACK, STANK BREATH ASSHOLES!"

If humans emitted sound effects for every movement executed, the sound of a car skidding would have been projected as the two teens rapidly turned around. Looking at each other, the teen that threatened the twins said something to the other, pulled out the gun, and both took off running after the boys. It was a wasted effort though. For as soon as the twins had blurted out their putdown, they took off like lightning for their building, and had more than enough distance to aid in their getaway...

"Keep running Shamel, no matter how tired you get!" Preacher huffed to Shamel.

"I know! I will! You keep running too!" Shamel huffed back.

The twins were almost at their building. They had been a little farther away than anticipated, but the adrenaline rush they built up from the incident kept them going, as they knew they would be safe at home.

Though out of breath and exhausted, like athletes nearing the finish line in a race, both Preacher and Shamel mustered up one last burst of energy and exploded through the tenement building door. The latch was broken, enabling it to swing open freely and forcefully. Rather than wait for the elevator and risk the two teen boys catching them, the twins hit the stairwell. They were startled by a group of six kids with their mother coming down the stairs, who all were equally as startled with the twins bounding up them. The twins continued on to the third floor where their apartment was. The boys didn't have keys, so they began to furiously pound on the door and call out, "Mom!" as loudly as they could. Though it seemed like an eternity for them, their mother opened the door rather quickly. She was holding the baby in her arms and fuming, then began to scold the twins…

"Where the hell have you two been? Did you go up on the roof? And why are you banging on this door like you have no sense?"

"Mom! Mom!" the twins pleaded.

"Shut up and get your 'tails' in here! I've told you about talking back..." Her voice trailed off for about two seconds, and then she began to yell even louder…"Shamel! Why are your pants wet? You couldn't hold it until you got home or at least find a tree?"

"Mom, -" Preacher began, but their mother abruptly cut him off…

"Shut up! I'm talking to your brother!"

"But Mom, -" Shamel began, and he too was abruptly cut off by their mother…

"SHUT-UP! Now I'm talking to **your** brother!"

Preacher felt desperate. He knew getting a word in edgewise wasn't going to be easy. So he just blurted out; "Some guy pulled a gun on us!"

Georgia's facial expression went from antagonism to disbelief…

"What? Somebody did what? She asked.

"Some guy pulled a gun on us, and that's why I peed on myself!" Shamel reiterated with despair.

Without wasting another moment, Georgia swooshed the boys into the apartment and slammed the door shut. After locking it, she went back to questioning them, but in a more nurturing and concerned tone of voice…

"Why did he pull a gun on you?"

"We don't know, mom! All that happened was I accidently bumped into him, then he pulled out his gun and was going to shoot me!" Shamel recapped, almost in tears.

"He was going to shoot me too, but his friend told him not to do it! And that's when we ran home, because they started chasing us!" Preacher concluded.

Georgia went and sat with the baby down on the sofa. She placed Venice next to her, then started wringing her hands together.

"Oh my God. Shamel, Preacher. No matter what it takes, I have to get this family out of the projects. I owe that to you, your sister, and whatever your new sibling to be is. Shamel, go get out of those clothes and wash up. Just put them in a plastic bag. Hopefully you both got a good look at those thugs, because I'm calling the police!"

As Shamel went to change, Preacher came and sat next to his baby sister on the sofa, while Georgia got on the phone and called 911.

Chapter Five

Henry, the twins' father arrived home from work after putting in some overtime. He stopped in the lobby of his building to check for mail from Saturday. Upon opening the box, he was delighted at receiving one letter in particular. He then stepped onto the elevator for the ride up to the third floor. The usual stench of urine didn't faze him this time, for he was as cheerful as he could be. Now as he stepped off the elevator, his nostrils were greeted with the smell of fried chicken. Henry optimistically hoped that smell was coming from his own apartment. Unfortunately, he was met with disharmony instead of a plate of hot food...

"Hi baby!" Henry cheerfully greeted Georgia with. Instead of greeting him back, she immediately informed him about what happened to the twins…

"Henry, I just finished talking with the Housing police before you came in. Do you know that some bastards pulled a gun on my babies?"

"Gun! What were they trying to do, rob them?" Henry asked very concerned, as he put his own firearm away.

"The way Shamel put it, these hoodlums just wanted to start trouble! I had to make him go wash up because he wet his clothes he was so frightened!"

Shamel, Preacher, and Venice were all sitting on the sofa. Shamel had a towel covering his legs to keep them warm. While Venice had a plastic cup, both he and Preacher were eating vanilla ice cream out of a bowl. Preacher looked up at his father and managed to brave a smile. Shamel put down his bowl of ice cream, got up and tightly hugged his father. Henry picked Shamel up and held him in his arms…

"Hey buddy. You ok?" Henry asked Shamel.

"Yes, dad. I'm sorry I wet my clothes." Shamel replied.

"Nothing to be ashamed of. You were scared. Were you scared too, Preacher?" the father asked.

"A little. I was *more mad* that they wouldn't let us say 'sorry' and leave."

"What happened exactly?"

"We were running home. Shamel bumped into the guy and apologized, but he pulled a gun anyway. His friend told him not to shoot us, and he didn't."

"But then they tried to sell us some drugs too!" Shamel added.

"Why didn't either you or Preacher tell me this before, Shamel? I would have told that to the police." their mother said.

"Sorry mom, I didn't think about it at the time." Shamel replied.

"We told them 'no' anyway!" Preacher declared proudly.

"Henry, I'm tired of living like this. Now I have to worry about the boys being killed by grown men over stupidity and trying to force drugs on them? Plus have to raise two more?" Georgia angrily demanded.

Henry put Shamel down, who still tried to cling to him. He handed Georgia the letter and said,

"I want you to read this."

"It's not the Health Department about their immunizations again, is it?" Georgia asked, irritated.

"No, just look."

Georgia looked at the mailing address on the front, then eagerly ripped it open and read the letter inside…

"Henry! You made it!" Georgia exclaimed, embracing him in a hug.

"That's right! The NYPD finally called me! Pretty soon, we'll be able to move out of the projects and into a house. A place that's bigger, -"

"Safer!" Georgia threw in, cutting him off. "You know, you may carry a gun already, but what good does that do us around here when you're not home? Then, if you shoot somebody **now**, they'll only try to burn you, because you're not in law enforcement!"

"I have Peace Officer status. But I was told from day one; 'If you're not protecting our money, you're not protected!' I'm all for the 'Officer Next Door' program, but I owe it to this family to be able to live in a safe and sound environment."

“We’re on the same page! It’s wonderful, because we have no idea if this one on the way is a single birth or another set of twins. And just an FYI, you’ve got a lot of nerve taking advantage of me when I was intoxicated.”

“That’s how we got the first set of twins, remember? You were sober with Venice.”

“Police or no police, no more babies!” Georgia scolded, then compassionately said, “I really am proud of you! Dinner’s ready. You can help me set the table.”

“What are we having?”

“Pork Chops with Black-eyed peas and Collard Greens.”

“Mmm. Reminds me of a joke. What’s the difference between a pig squealing, and a rat squealing?”

“I don’t know. How you pull the tail?”

“No. The Mafia doesn’t go after pigs!”

“Crazy!” Georgia replied, giggling. That made the boys laugh too, especially Shamel.

“Any ice cream for dessert?” Henry asked.

"No. The twins were so upset; I let them and their sister finish the rest. I'll bake you some cinnamon rolls." Georgia answered.

She kissed Henry on the cheek, then they both went into the kitchen area to put the dinner plates together. Shamel sat back down on the sofa next to Preacher again.

"I'm glad daddy's home." Shamel said to Preacher.

"Me too. I hope we never see those guys again, either!" Preacher replied.

"Well, when I grow up, I want to bust them! Like in 'New Jack City'!"

"Oooh, you *was* looking at daddy's *bootleg*!"

"So were you! You know we're too young to get into movies like that!"

"Well, I *wanna* bust them too. Cause this is our 'New Jack City' and we have to defend it!"

"Word!" Shamel agreed, as he and Preacher gave each other a hi-five.

"Boys, bring your sister and come sit and eat." their father spoke aloud.

Soon the entire family was seated. They gave *grace,* and began enjoying their meal.

Chapter Six

The next day at work, Henry's eagerness about being called by the NYPD was still apparent, as he displayed a broad smile. His co-workers decided to tease him…

"Hey Henry, got *some* this morning?" Baron queried.

"Yeah, the only other time you smile like that is when it's payday!" Monroe chimed in.

"Oh, I've got a reason to smile. Pretty soon you two will be training some rookie how to walk, chew gum, and carry money bags at the same time." Henry replied.

There was a brief silence, as Baron and Monroe gave Henry an inquisitive look. Then Monroe said, "Oh hell, he's gonna rob the truck! You could've let me in on it, you know!"

"That's right! We can grab at least one bag each, since we'll have to cover for you as you make your way out of the country!" Baron added.

Henry laughed wholeheartedly…

"You guys are crazy! I wouldn't..."

"That new job with the police department come through?" Monroe blurted out before Henry could finish.

"Yes!" Henry enthusiastically replied.

"Congratulations, you traitor!" Baron jokingly said.

"Thanks! I will miss you guys though." Henry said.

"So when's the party?" Baron asked.

"We can go out for beers this weekend. But it's still a love affair, guys. I won't be leaving for at least three months." Henry said.

"No good! You've got to go now! It'll only make things harder!" joked Monroe.

"Tell you what, after this run, you two can treat me to breakfast. And I don't mean some damn bagel either!" replied Henry.

Monroe countered, "Oh, listen to him! He wants eggs and grits, -"

"And toast and juice!" - Henry butted in.

"Look. All I had this morning was saliva, so can we quit talking about food and go enjoy some when we finish?" Baron jokingly scoffed. Tragically however, this was to be their last morning together sharing such camaraderie…

Henry pulled up in front of their first pick up location, which was a Savings and Loan. Following standard procedure, Monroe got out first, drew his weapon, and walked around to the back of the armored truck. After assessing all was clear, he tapped on the rear door of the truck to notify Baron. Baron got out and entered the S&L, while Henry stayed behind the wheel. Once Baron emerged from the S&L with the deposits, Monroe tapped on the rear of the truck again, signaling that all was clear. But no sooner had he turned the key in the lock to open the rear doors, that they were attacked. Seemingly out of nowhere, five masked gunmen emerged. Monroe screamed, **"AMBUSH!"** – Though his weapon was already drawn, he was fired upon immediately with shots striking him in the chest, abdomen area, and left leg, and unable to defend himself. While his vest did stop the upper body rounds, the bullet that struck his leg hit the femoral artery, sealing his fate on the scene.

Baron also screamed out, **"AMBUSH!"** – and dropping the currency bags, immediately pulled out his weapon and began firing, striking one of the gunmen in the chest. Henry flung open the driver's side door of the armored truck in an attempt to rescue Baron. But before Baron could climb in, another gunman shot him in the back of his neck. Baron fell backwards off the step of the truck and lay motionless, with his eyes wide open. Henry yelled out, "BARON!", but got no response. Pulling his own weapon, Henry popped out the driver's side door and shot the same gunman that felled Baron. That left only three gunmen to battle. Henry then slid across the bench seat of the armored truck and out the passenger side where he confronted and shot another gunman fatally in his chest. Stepping towards the engine and using the passenger door as a shield, Henry traded shots with the fourth gunman, striking him in the chest, shoulder, and arm. That left only one. Unfortunately, while Henry was battling it out with the gunman he'd just shot, the last gunman managed to sneak around to the driver's side of the truck, which still had the door open. Henry climbed back up into the passenger side of the truck with the intent of barricading himself inside until help could arrive - and was blasted right in the head by the last gunman.

At the memorial service, Henry was lauded as a hero, and being interred with full military honors. The priest gave some final words of comfort. But while Georgia sat holding Venice, with Preacher and Shamel on both sides of her, Shamel got up and walked over to the casket. First, he touched it. Then as the Honor Guard gave their 21-gun salute, Shamel bent over the coffin, laid his head in his arms, and began to wail. Shot. Cry. Shot. Cry. Shot. Cry. Shot… -- and Shamel jumped out of his sleep. He was sweating and mildly hyperventilating. His cell phone alarm was going off and it was pretty loud. Subconsciously, the shots from the 21-gun salute in his dream resembled the sound effect from the song he chose as a ringtone, which was 'Play at your own risk' by *Planet Patrol*. Shamel turned off the alarm, then continued to lie in bed for about 15 extra minutes to compose himself. Finally he got up to prepare for his day. After quickly freshening up in the bathroom and dressing, Shamel hurried off to work. He didn't have far to travel, but nevertheless couldn't stand being late.

Chapter Seven

B.L.I.N.G.

As per the NYPD, the acronym stands for:

Bringing **L**ong **I**ncarceration to **N**arcotics **G**angs.

Ironically, it was a convicted drug dealer who inspired the idea. During the penalty phase of a particular trial, the Assistant District Attorney was giving his closing statement…

"Here before you, ladies and gentlemen of the jury, sits one of the most violent and unremorseful drug dealers I've ever had the pleasure and responsibility of having put away. Just ask the surviving members of the 'Trower' family. Ask them what they have had to endure over the past year and a half. The brutal execution style murders of both sets of grandparents, who weren't even involved in this mess. The violent murder of the pregnant aunt and her two young children; – babies! The sexual assault and killing of the girlfriend of his rival. And finally, the killing of his rival – the true intended target. But instead of just shooting him like he did the others, he wanted to send a message. Set an example. So he hacks off his nemesis' private part – with a serrated knife, and puts it in a bag of empty crack vials. Never in my entire career as a prosecutor have I come across someone more vile than this dealer. I think his 'Honor' will agree with me, that no sentence is truly good or long enough. But I would much rather have him rot in prison, than be loose to commit such an atrocity ever again. All this talk about 'bling, bling'. What on earth does 'bling' stand for anyway? No further comments."

"Mr. Charles, any final words before I impose sentencing?" the Judge asked.

The Dealer stood up and spoke…

"Yeah, I got some final words. You wanna know what 'bling' represents? What 'bling' stands for? In my case, 'bling' stands for 'Being Locked-up Indefinitely with No Grease!' This system sucks!"

The judge hit his gavel on the sound block and admonished the dealer…

"Order in my courtroom!"

"Screw your court, and this sentencing hearing! I want a rematch! Retrial! Whatever!" the dealer proclaimed in an angry outburst.

"Bailiff, secure and remand the defendant to custody! As for you Mr. Charles, you are hereby sentenced to…"

Amid all the commotion from the sudden outburst, the police officers that were present at the hearing began to talk among themselves. Something the dealer said struck a chord. After a small brainstorming session, and with the blessing of top police brass, the District Attorneys and the Mayor, they took the negative connotation of 'bling' that the dealer implied, and turned it into a positive permanent fixture in the NYPD's war on drugs.

The precinct is brand new. Nestled in the 'Sugar Hill' section of Manhattan, B.L.I.N.G. was a welcome addition to the neighborhood. Much like the United States Marine Corps is under the Department of the Navy; B.L.I.N.G.'s structure is moored by the same ideology, as the unit is under the NYPD's Organized

Crime Control Bureau's gang division. Its inception was initially met with resistance as Internal Affairs and the New York Civil Liberties Union argued that no one unit should have so much autonomy, especially in the ongoing battle against corruption. While the number of undercover officers assigned to narcotics is low in general, B.L.I.N.G. detectives helped keep the arrests of drug suspects at a healthy level. The law enforcers assigned to B.L.I.N.G. were coming up with such impressive numbers in apprehending all level drug suspects, eventually the naysayers backed off and allowed B.L.I.N.G. to coexist as an independent entity. That was important in order for the unit to receive federal subsidization. This is one of the factors that sets B.L.I.N.G. apart from the regular narcotics division. For one, B.L.I.N.G. personnel receive higher pay than other NYPD units. Another factor is the region they have jurisdiction over. In conjunction with the Drug Enforcement Administration, B.L.I.N.G. detectives cover all of New York State. This is the reason why getting assigned to B.L.I.N.G. isn't easy. As mentioned earlier, B.L.I.N.G. is modeled after the USMC. The detectives make up the 'grunts' or ground units. The uniformed officers in ranking from Sergeants up to the Chief of the Department make up the logistics and intelligence team. The few patrol officers that are assigned handle functions such as manning police lines and barricades during active crime scenes, as well as perimeter security during raids. All detectives who are chosen for B.L.I.N.G. must agree to longer than normal work hours. That's in addition to being on call 24 hours a day. Vacation and personal time off could be overridden based on the need for manpower, especially during planned raids. And though there are methods of faking sampling, there would be situations when a detective would have to ingest some drugs to avoid blowing their cover, if not save their own life. Still, B.L.I.N.G. has some of the most dedicated law enforcers in the department.

Tour II (the day shift) was Shamel's regular shift. As he was on his way inside the precinct, he encountered one of his co-workers from Tour I on the way out…

"Hey papa, *you* kinda late!"

"*S'up*, Angel! How was the night shift?" Shamel replied.

"It was a slow night. The most excitement my partner and I had? Some guy who ran a red light. Aside from the fact he did it right in front of us, we were bored, so we pulled him over. Turns out he had a suspended license, no insurance, -"

"And warrants?" Shamel asked enthusiastically.

"Nah, we couldn't get that lucky! But we did give him hell for the small amount of weed he had in his possession! Believe me when I say we had a ball calling the tow truck to impound his vehicle!" Angel boasted.

"Ha! Wish I had been there! But let me get on in. Have a good night, day, however you sleep!"

"You have a safe tour. By the way, I heard you haven't been getting your recommended daily allowance of crap, so I left some 'Ex-Lax' on your desk."

"I don't know where you heard that crap from, but you can kiss my *Grande culo*!" Shamel scolded.

"That would be a **whole** lot of kissing, Papa!" Angel retorted.

Shamel just laughed as they waved good bye to one another and he continued inside. Shamel's co-workers on the day shift were a very jovial bunch. Roll call was always upbeat, with the staff acting more like young college freshmen than mature adults. It's not that they were unprofessional; they just knew how to have fun…

The Tour Commander spoke up in a loud, clear tone of voice,

"All right, quiet down and listen for your family, birth, government, or stage name, whatever turns you on. You all know the procedure. Either answer when I call your name…"

"**Or give you our pay for the day!**" the entire room bellowed out loud in unison.

The Tour Commander continued...

"Starline!"

"I did not have sexual relations with that blow-up doll!" he answered.

"Uh, sure you didn't! 'Harmon'!"

"It was *da* 'Warriors'!" Harmon responded.

"Flynn!"

"All right, *ya doity* rats!" Flynn responded.

"By the way, 'Flynn' there's an adjustment check for you." (Someone in the background griped, "What about me?" The Tour Commander ignored it and called the next name...)

"Dalton!"

"At-ti-ca! At-ti-ca!" came the response.

"Russell!"

"Ri-kers! Ri-kers!" came that response.

"Davis!"

"To the Bat Poles! No, make that the stripper poles!" he responded.

"All right, calm it down. Remember we have women working here too." the Tour Commander admonished before continuing...

"Charms!"

"President." - - a soft but audible female voice called out.

"Haynes!"

"Better late than never!" – Shamel declared as he walked in the room just as his name was called.

"Know what? Just for you, I'm going to alphabetize the list!" the Tour Commander chided.

"Aw *Sarge,* then I won't be able to stop at 'Krispy Kreme' anymore!" Shamel exclaimed, to a room full of laughter. The woman with the soft voice scowled at Shamel as he made his way towards the center of the group, but she didn't say a word to him. The Tour Commander continued…

"Parker-Green!"

"Lucy, *ju* got some *'splaining* to do!" a voice replied.

"Ferguson, better known as Viper!"

"Protected by 'Viper' – **Stand back!**" – the entire room answered along with him.

"Weich!" the Tour Commander continued.

"In the flesh!" he answered.

"O'Brannon!"

"Vacation in one day!" - a woman replied.

"You better hope it's not **<u>one</u>** day! Good for you! 'Steele'!" – the Tour Commander continued.

"On vacation!" someone yelled out. The Tour Commander noted it and called the next name.

"Everett!"

"Ask not what your precinct can do for you!" came his answer.

"Laconi!"

"Modified duty!" – a burly Caucasian male leaning on the wall in the back with his arms folded shouted out in a less than cheerful tone of voice. The entire room became silent, as everyone turned to look at him. The Tour Commander shook his head as he logged the man's attendance.

"You know the rules. No street assignments during an internal investigation. Ok, who's left?" the Tour Commander continued…

"Zhao!"

"*Me* Chinese, *me* play joke…"

"That's why I drink 'Pepsi'." the Tour Commander responded. Continuing on…

"Robinson!"

"Now on maternity leave!" someone else yelled out.

"When did she give birth?" the sergeant asked.

"At 3am this morning. It's a boy! I already have a card for her." the same person answered again.

"Wonderful! Pass it around the entire department, and make sure everyone signs it. I will have some flowers and balloons ordered for her." the sergeant said, before continuing with the roster.

"Lamb! (a pause). Lamb!"

"Out sick." someone again yelled out.

"And finally, 'Cunningham', who I already know is on a stakeout. Good Morning, Tour two!"

"Good Morning, Sergeant Zanzabar!" the entire room responded together.

"Before we get down to official business, I want all of you to extend a warm welcome to the newest member of *our Justice League…*" Sergeant Zanzabar said, gesturing to a woman who had been standing next to the podium since the start of roll call. "This is detective Lavender Divine."

"Hi, Detective Divine!" the room bellowed out.

"Detective Divine, you'll be partnering with 'Viper'." the Tour Commander instructed.

"Cool." she replied, as she went and stood next to him. She also made eye contact and smiled at Detective Charms, who nodded her head and smiled back.

The rest of roll call was basic daily information the detectives received. Sergeant Zanzabar, began to wrap up…

"Congratulations are in order for 'Viper' who made 'Detective of the Quarter'!"

The room broke out in applause.

"And though there are no consolation prizes, 'Shamel' receives honorable mention for being a close runner up! All of you do great work, and I know it will continue!"

"Please, no applause!" Shamel joked.

"Glory Hound!" Detective Charms said.

Sergeant Zanzabar motioned for the room to quiet down again…

"One final item. On a sad note, you're all aware that the NYPD lost one of its own from a Brooklyn unit last night. Details of the memorial service and where donations can be sent will be available via the *Intranet*, as well as the bulletin board and the 99th precinct's webpage. As always, you're all encouraged to attend. Like I always say, this could be <u>your</u> last tour, - so put God first on your shift. That's all."

There was a low murmur as everyone began to partner up and disperse. The detective on modified duty noisily exited the room while muttering under his breath. Detective Charms walked up to Shamel, made a fist with her left hand and punched him on the arm…

"Owww!" Shamel exclaimed as he reacted by drawing up and making a pitiful face.

"Late night again?"

"Oh, cut me some slack, Sequoia! I went to bed at a decent hour!" Shamel replied, crossing his fingers behind his back.

Sequoia peeked behind him, and upon catching his fingers crossed, exclaimed, "Later for you, 'Rip Van Winkle'! Anyway, I want to formerly introduce you to Lavender! She's the one I've been telling you about!"

Sequoia said enthusiastically. Sequoia walked up to Viper and Detective Divine who were conversing with each other.

"Lavender, it's great to see and be working with you again!" she said to her.

"I know! I'm so happy!" Lavender replied, as she and Sequoia hugged each other.

Sequoia motioned for Shamel to come closer, and then explained, "Lavender and I were in the academy together, but after graduation, we were assigned to different precincts."

"You're so lucky to have 'Viper' for a partner. Want to trade?" Shamel chuckled, as he nudged Sequoia.

"Shamel's being modest. If you have any questions and I'm not around, he's the man to go to!" Viper responded.

"And you're not getting rid of me! Just for that comment, you're buying lunch!" Sequoia challenged Shamel.

"Just curious, what made you leave 'Special Victims Unit'?" Shamel asked Lavender.

"I couldn't take it!" Lavender replied, exasperated. She continued, "All those unsolved sexual assaults. Rape kits on top of rape kits. What finally put me over the edge is this latest string of attacks solely against non-English speaking women."

"They'll catch that punk. In any case, welcome aboard!" Shamel answered, extending his hand to shake Lavender's.

Lavender looked at Shamel's hand and said, "I thought *we was' fam'*. You better give me a hug and act like you really want me here!"

"Ah, suki-suki! Group hug!" Shamel yelled out. Upon that, he, Sequoia, Lavender, and Viper all hugged.

"Told you she was cool *peoples*! Sequoia hummed.

"Hey, Sequoia mentioned that you have a twin brother on the force. Any chance of meeting him?" Lavender asked Shamel.

"Well, he's actually a detective in Virginia. But hey, anything's possible. Don't ask me why, but I have a feeling you'll all be meeting him in the near, distant future."

Upon that, the four of them went to get their assignments and breakfast to start their day.

Chapter Eight

The weatherman said it would be a balmy 81 degrees and sunny, without too much humidity. Good day to wash the SUV, as indicated by the long line extending around the corner from the car wash. On the exit side, the sunlight glistening off the beads of water caught the attention of two sexy black women walking by. Maybe it was the Deep Cherry Red Crystal Pearl color of the Jeep Grand Cherokee. Maybe it was the handsome black male standing off to the side, waiting for the Jeep to be dried off. In any case, the two women stopped and looked admiringly at the black male in a somewhat flirtatious pose. The man smiled at both women, then sheepishly raised his left hand which was holding his cell phone to display the platinum wedding band on his finger. In a flustered tone, one of the women looked at the other and commented as they both hurried on their way,

"See! All the good ones are taken!"

"Yeah, but who said **he** was any good?" the other replied, defiantly.

The man just smiled and sighed as he watched them leave. By that time, the Jeep was fully out the wash and being wiped down by an attendant. At that moment, the man's cell phone rang. Without glancing at the caller ID, he tapped the screen and spoke…

"Hey Claudine. (Purr)."

"(Giggle) Preacher, what are you doing?"

"Finishing up at the car wash!" Preacher cheerfully replied. He then began to scrutinize the wash job, but had a very pleasant disposition over the outcome of his nitpicking…

"Wow! Pascual did a slamming job with that simonize compound, getting rid of those blemishes. This thing looks showroom new!" he thought to himself.

This was Detective Preacher Haynes – Shamel's identical twin. They both liked staying groomed with a goatee and mustache, sometimes with a razor line connecting the beard. What distinguished the two of them was their piercings, as Preacher wore a diamond in each ear, while Shamel sported a cross in both of his.

Preacher was a law enforcer assigned with the Alexandria, Virginia police unit; D. E. T. E. R. - (Drug Enforcement Task Emergency Reconnaissance). He was off duty, but had agreed to do a favor for a fellow officer by delivering some paperwork to an insurance claims adjuster's office, after which he was heading home to be with his family…

"So are we going to 'Maryland House' for dinner?"

"Um, yeah. Hold on Claudine…" Preacher's voice trailed off as he reached into his pocket and pulled out a five dollar bill to give to the attendant who had completed drying off the Jeep. He handed the attendant his tip and said "Thanks Pascual", before resuming his conversation on the cell phone… "You're getting lazy on me. How come you don't want to cook?"

"Look here *Chef Boy-R-Feed;* it was you who promised the kids and me dinner. Ain't no Betty Wright around telling me to be a cook in the kitchen, not tonight!"

"True, but Taco Bell is free on Tuesday's for kids. Free!" Preacher replied, snickering.

"Yeah, ok. You gonna end up hurt and hungry. I'll just haul the kids off to Inner Harbor alone, and leave you to fend for yourself!" Claudine huffed.

Preacher climbed into the Jeep, shifted into gear and drove off. He went down Route 1 towards Fairfax County, still discussing dinner with Claudine…

"C'mon baby, you know my money's been acting funny."

"Sure, ever since you met me, right?"

"No, I'm just saying, 'Bro-man' ain't been getting no overtime lately.(Chortling) Looks like the 'Commonwealth' and I ain't got *no* wealth in common!"

"Cheap Bastard!" Claudine replied, laughing along with Preacher.

"Hey, I'm just kidding. Of course I'm still taking all of you out. But it's only 2:55 in the afternoon, so *why you* stressing me?" Preacher asked.

"I've learned to put my bids in early with you, 'Car 54'. Why do you think I'm always asking where you at?" Claudine replied.

"All right, I've told you *'bout* calling me out my name, - Hey!"

Preacher abruptly hit his brakes and stopped his conversation as a late model Cutlass Supreme came careening around the corner with tires squealing just when the traffic signal for its direction changed from green to red. Preacher let down his power window and yelled out after them, "You wanna try slowing down?" The car pulled in front of a 'Crispus Attucks Federal Credit Union' branch and stopped. At first, Preacher was indifferent to it all for he kept driving. But something told him that things weren't right with this scenario. He made a U-turn, headed back towards the intersection where the car came speeding from...

"Claudine, I have to go but I'll call you back."

"Is everything all right?" Claudine asked.

"Yeah baby, but I have to go right now. I'll call you back, I promise."

"Okay, I love you. Be careful."

"I will, Love you too. Bye."

Preacher ended the call. Now he was sitting on the adjacent corner behind the Cutlass. Patiently, he watched the credit union and noted the time which was 2:57.

"Maybe they just had to get there before it closed." Preacher thought to himself, though he didn't actually believe it. After being in law enforcement for some time, one develops crime intuition. It's the same as street smarts - but more focused on criminal activity. His cop acumen paid off. Though he hadn't noticed anyone enter the credit union initially because he kept driving, Preacher observed someone in the driver's seat of the Cutlass, and then saw one, two, three - and a fourth man exit the branch. All four were wearing ball caps and sunglasses. The first two men had backpacks which appeared bulky. The third man was carrying a canvas sack — the kind financial institutions use. The fourth and last man had a shotgun with a pistol grip in plain view. At that same moment a call came over Preacher's police radio…

"Attention all units in the vicinity of Crystal and Pentagon cities, 10–90 received from the 'Crispus Attucks Federal Credit Union' on Route 1, please respond…"

As the last man exited the credit union, he turned around and fired the shotgun into the doors of the branch, before jumping in the back seat of the Cutlass Supreme. Once his door slammed shut, the Cutlass took off with tires squealing - and Preacher took off right behind them! The Cutlass picked up speed as it headed towards the interstate on Route 1. Preacher steadily applied the gas in an attempt to keep up with the car. He flipped down his red flasher, turned on his dazzle lights and siren and got on his handheld police radio…

"This is Detective Haynes, Alexandria police, responding to that silent alarm. I'm now pursuing a late model blue Cutlass Supreme with Virginia plates, westbound on Route 1. Approximately five assailants including the driver. Suspects armed and dangerous. Shots fired. I say again, shots fired. Requesting immediate backup."

Preacher's police radio came alive with various law enforcement responses. The voice of a female dispatcher came back first…

"10-4. All units, Detective Haynes requiring assistance with a 10–80, westbound on Route 1."

"This is Trooper Donville with the Virginia State police. I'm in the vicinity of Route 1, on my way to assist."

"This is Lieut. Eesaa with the Virginia State police. I want Virginia DOT and all available State units on traffic patrol to shut down those HOV lanes North and South of 95 and 395 immediately!"

"This is Lieut. Merriweather with DC Metro police. We have units on standby at Interstate 295 leading to Pennsylvania Avenue ready to intercept. Be careful, Preacher."

"10-4, Lieut." Preacher responded.

Preacher drove with conviction – he was determined to get these armed robbers! As soon as both vehicles passed Army-Navy Drive, the state trooper that responded first joined the chase…

"I'm right behind you, Detective!" trooper Donville radioed to Preacher.

Preacher didn't reply, as both of his hands tightly gripped the steering wheel for better control of the SUV. The suspects in the Cutlass weren't the least bit thrilled at all with this new development. The one in the back seat with the shotgun fired a shot out the back passenger window into the air, then another at both pursuing vehicles. Preacher quickly got back on his handheld radio…

"I've got more shots fired! They're shooting at us now!"

"Preacher, break off the chase! Don't get yourself killed!" - a voice rumbled back through the handheld radio. It was Preacher's commanding officer.

"I got this, chief!" Preacher responded back.

He did back off slightly after the shotgun blast and tried to maintain a safe distance, but that's when trooper Donville decided to take over the lead. For the most part, traffic was light westbound on Route 1 which enabled the chase to occur. But headed southbound towards Route 1, was an ambulance with its own emergency lights and siren on. In general, it's hard to decipher the direction an emergency vehicle is coming from when it's at a distance. However, when there is more than one emergency vehicle headed towards the same point, it's nearly impossible to determine direction and distance of both. Disaster was only an RPM away…

Trooper Donville sped up and passed Preacher.

"I'll try to ram them!" he spoke into his radio.

"No!" Preacher yelled into his own radio. "Too much risk invo-"

Preacher didn't even get a chance to finish his sentence. Apparently at that moment neither the trooper nor the driver of the ambulance was aware of the other's presence. The Cutlass blew through the intersection against a red light. The ambulance which had a clear lane of traffic and the right-of-way with a green light, proceeded to go through the intersection as well when it was struck in the rear by trooper Donville's cruiser. The ambulance lost control, and flipped onto its side. Trooper Donville spun out of control as well, and slammed into some parked vehicles in front of an apartment building. Preacher who was already at a distance hit his brakes and swerved to avoid the scattered debris in his path. As he passed the accident and looked at the aftermath in his rearview mirror, he declared out loud, "This has to end now!"

It seemed Preacher was finally about to get a break. Traffic had built up on the interstate due to it being rush-hour, and from the closure of the HOV lanes. The driver of the Cutlass decided to look for an alternate route, and turned onto Eisenhower Avenue. That proved to be all of the suspected offenders undoing, as well as the beginning to the end of the high-speed chase. Eisenhower Avenue was a direct route towards the Pentagon. On the grounds of the Pentagon itself, more law enforcement personnel were present than usual. That's because the Vice President and Joint Chiefs of Staff had just lifted off in Marine One, - the big green military presidential helicopter. Because of barricades as well as structural design, the Cutlass had nowhere to go but straight; and it ran into the wrought iron fence of the Pentagon while Marine One was still literally hovering just a few feet off the ground. First came the loud squeal of breaks, then the awful sound of metal crushing into metal before the Cutlass came to halt. At that same instant, a blast from the shotgun was heard, then there was silence. Preacher pulled up a few feet behind the Cutlass, shut off his siren, opened his door and drew his firearm through the window. Other law enforcement units that had responded were pulling up as well. But in addition to the state police and local units from Alexandria and Arlington that came to render assistance, the suspects had to deal with Pentagon personnel; – Army, Navy, Air Force, Marine security guards in their dress uniforms, and of course the Secret Service. While the fence had sustained damage, it was still intact. All of the Pentagon personnel with firearms had them drawn; from 9 mm handguns and M-16 A2 rifles to automatic submachine guns; everyone's weapon was now trained on the Cutlass. A tourist might have mistaken this for some movie shoot. But it was all very real and frightening. After the terror attacks of September 11, 2001, no one took anything lightly, especially if it involved a perceived attack or threat against a government installation.

Preacher yelled out to the occupants of the Cutlass, "Ride's over! I want the driver to exit first! Throw out any weapons you have! Open your door slowly, keep your hands visible, and lay on the ground!"

There was no response, no movement at all. Suddenly without warning, the back door on the right passenger side opened. The man with the shotgun came out and fired towards the fence of the Pentagon. Pellets from the blast struck one of the naval staff members, turning his work whites into a red splattered blood mosaic. The gunman then tried to make a run for it, but was fatally cut down by armed Pentagon personnel who unmercifully and unrelentingly opened fire on him. Preacher just shook his head as he looked at the suspect crumpled on the ground. Preacher now cautiously emerged from behind the door of the Jeep, staying low as he approached the Cutlass. This time, figuring that the front seat occupants were probably unconscious, he issued a different command…

"You in the backseat on the driver's side! Throw your weapon out the window, keep your hands where I can see them and exit the vehicle!"

The man in the backseat complied, first tossing a gun out the window, then groggily spilling out of the backseat onto the ground.

"Hands outstretched in front of you, palms down!" Preacher barked at him. "Next man, in the middle seat! Throw out your weapon, and get on the ground!"

"He's dead. So's the guy in the front passenger seat." the man already on the ground wearily said to Preacher.

What had occurred; as the man with the shotgun was reloading it, he was jarred when the car hit the fence. The shotgun went off at point-blank range right into the middle suspect's torso. The suspect riding in the front passenger seat slammed into the windshield upon impact with the fence, breaking his neck in the process. That left the driver…

"Don't you move!" Preacher ordered the man lying on the ground.

"We've got him covered!" one of the Pentagon's military personnel shouted to Preacher.

Now Preacher shouted again for the driver to exit…

"I can't open my door! It's jammed! I'll climb out the window!" the driver yelled back."

"Keep your hands where I can see them, and come out of the car slowly!" Preacher responded.

This time however when Preacher told the man to exit, he overlooked the command to throw out any weapons. That would prove to be critical. The driver finally exited the Cutlass, stumbling as his feet hit the ground. He turned around, withdrew a gun from his waistband and put it to his own head, then backed up against the fence next to the totaled Cutlass. Now came the showdown. All of the Pentagon personnel were yelling at him to drop his gun. The entire police backup was yelling at him to drop his gun including Preacher. The suspect was yelling back, threatening to take his own life…

"I'll do it! I'll kill myself! I swear I will!"

Preacher held up his left hand signaling the Pentagon personnel to back off which they did. He slowly approached the suspect, still taking heed to the one lying on the ground.

"Listen," Preacher began. "You saw what happened to your boy with the shotgun. Personally, I don't care if you kill yourself or not. But just in case you're dubious, I'll help you!"

Preacher raised his weapon and pointed it at the suspect's head. "We're not going to stand here for the rest of the afternoon and call in hostage negotiators for a suicidal *perp* looking for freedom. Either you give yourself up, or I'll see to it that Georgetown University's medical program gets another cadaver, courtesy of the Alexandria, Police!"

The suspect still held his gun to his head. Preacher still aimed his weapon at the suspect's head. All of the Pentagon personnel and responding law enforcers kept their weapons trained on both suspects. It seemed like hours, but after about four minutes and Preacher uttering, "What's it going to be?" it was over. The suspect slowly lowered his gun, then dropped it on the ground and broke down crying. Uniformed Alexandria police officers moved in to make the arrest of both suspects. Only after they were handcuffed did all of the law enforcers at the scene holster or shoulder their weapons. Some ran over to the sailor who had been shot. A news helicopter which had been monitoring the police frequency was hovering above, and caught the entire incident on video from the time to chase was in progress. Preacher knew that meant he was going to have to be ready to face the media once he returned to the precinct. Walking back over to the Jeep, Preacher stopped short and groaned out loud. A few of the pellets from the earlier shotgun blast had struck the SUV, ruining the finish.

"Pascual is going to be madder than I am!" Preacher kidded aloud to himself. He then got on his police radio…"Detective Haynes to dispatch…"

"Dispatch, go ahead."

"10–95 at the Pentagon. Unfortunately, we do have persons requiring medical attention. Requesting 10-52. Scene is secure."

"10-4, Detective Haynes. EMS units in route."

A police officer with the Arlington PD recognized Preacher and shouted over to him, "Hey Preach! You okay?"

Preacher looked over and responded, "Yeah, Melvin! I'm just fine, thanks."

Preacher looked at the clock in his dash. It was 3:36 pm. A whole hour hadn't even passed, and all this drama went down. He wondered to himself if he would still be able to take Claudine and the kids out to dinner. With the amount of paperwork he was going to have to process behind this incident, Preacher figured he'd be lucky to get a hot dog from '7-Eleven'.

Chapter Nine

It was a dark and stormy night… No, seriously. Preacher called Claudine back as he promised and explained the incident to her. Claudine wasn't happy about Preacher having been in such a dangerous situation, but she was used to it by now. She also would rather hear it from Preacher himself than on the evening news…

"Don't worry about the kids and myself. If you like, I can prepare something now and keep your plate warm, or we'll just order pizza."

"I'll try to get out of here as soon as I can. We may still be able to go out tonight." Preacher replied.

"Don't promise me a Rolls-Royce, then hand me a bicycle! You know I hate that." Claudine haughtily admonished.

"I'm going to handle my *biz* quick, then get with you and our crumb-snatchers."

"Watch what you say about my children." Claudine chastised without being serious.

"Dag-nabbit! They're my tax credits too! Anyway, I'll call back if I get stuck."

"Please do, and I love you – sometimes!"

"Love you too, Dini. Bye."

"Bye."

Both Preacher and Claudine hung up simultaneously.

The precinct was bustling with activity in light of the spectacular chase and capture of the credit union hold up gang. A media camp had been set up outside for a press conference. The actual arresting officers were processing the two remaining suspects. Preacher was glad, for he knew that meant he would get home a lot faster. Preacher headed to the locker room to take a quick shower and change clothes. Upon entering, other officers were slapping him high-fives, as well as on his back and congratulating him on a job well done. The talk was excited and high energy, even for officers that were not involved in the chase. Everyone was trying to evaluate and compare notes on the arrest…

"If that were my truck, I would have rammed them!" one cop said.

"And mess up my front end? *S'matter* with you? Preacher guffawed, as he opened his locker.

"I think you handled your business, Detective!" another cop yelled out. But just as Preacher was about to respond to that comment, the room became hushed. An older, distinguished looking gentleman entered the locker room. He was a husky white male with salt and pepper hair as well as a matching thick mustache. His face was chiseled, with no visible wrinkles. He also had a stern look about him. In a firm tone of voice he said, "Preacher, in my office."

Preacher immediately closed his locker and followed the man out of the locker room. A low murmur could be heard as the other officers looked on and quietly talked amongst themselves....

"So, when did you move from narcotics to robbery squad?" the man asked Preacher, as the two of them walked down the corridor.

"I just so happened to be in the right place at the wrong time?" Preacher modestly questioned.

As the man and Preacher entered an office, the man said to Preacher, "Have a seat." upon which Preacher did after closing the door behind them. The office was spacious and well lit. Though most were commendations, various awards decorated the room, both on the walls and on shelves. In one corner stood an American flag, as well as the flag of the Commonwealth of Virginia and the flag of the City of Alexandria. The desk was tidy. On it were two small picture frames with photos of the man's family. On one corner were some neatly stacked documents. A pen holder, letter opener, telephone, pencil sharpener, paperweight, coffee mug and police scanner also took up space on the desk. A gold plated nameplate on the desk read, 'Chief Dan Fortson'. In the center of the desk, was a small bowl of pralines. As the man walked around the desk to his chair, he gestured to the pralines with his hand, offering some to Preacher who obliged. The man didn't sit in the chair however, opting to sit instead on a free corner of his desk. Preacher was a bit anxious. He had no idea why he was called into the office, but figured he would entertain the thought…

"Am I here to be commended on another job well done, chief?" Preacher asked earnestly.

The chief clasped his hands together, looked Preacher right in his eyes and said in a non-enthused tone of voice, "I know you were solicited by the DEA."

Preacher's mouth dropped open. He hung his head down and in a low tone of voice replied, "Oh." Preacher's embarrassment was apparent. He looked back up at Chief Fortson and said, "If it makes a difference, I still have to go back for a second round of interviews."

After a brief silence, Chief Fortson spoke… "What is it with this unit?" he asked, getting up from the edge of the desk and walking over to the window. "I lose more guys through attrition than to line of duty injuries, not that I want to see my officers hurt of course." Chief Fortson turned to Preacher and pondered, "Am I that bad of a leader?"

Preacher shifted in the chair to make himself more comfortable. He looked at the chief and said, "Chief, you're not a bad leader at all. I can't speak for the entire unit, but I've always wanted to work for the DEA. I know morale is high, if not above average. I just think, well, this unit is too slow for most of the cops that join it."

The chief walked back to the desk and sat on the edge again. "Preacher, you're the best detective in this department. I'm not just saying that. But the retention rate for officers here has been terrible. When I heard you were possibly leaving as well, I felt very disappointed. Hassaan was the only other detective in this unit I thought I could count on to show the new crop how the veterans handled things. Next thing I know, he runs off to the West Coast and joins the LAPD."

"True, but in his defense, he only went because he's chasing behind that movie star girlfriend of his." Preacher said, and in a low whisper added, "Hell, I would!"

"I don't know, Preacher. I still get the impression that I'm too hard on the troops. Crime in our district is down 60%. Now where else in America have you heard a comparable number? Not even the major cities like New York, Chicago, Detroit, and Boston can boast of such success! However, we have that number largely because I spearheaded the effort to make my officers more accountable, in addition to increasing the ranks. I can't stress enough, the pride and attention to detail I require of the men and women working here. Yet it seems that no one stays long enough for the appreciation to truly set in."

Preacher took another handful of pralines, but stopped short of putting them in his mouth…

"Tell you what, chief. You don't have long until retirement, right?"

"I still have a few good years left. Two, three at the most." the chief replied.

"I'll make a deal with you. I will stay until you retire. This way, I can help bring up that 60% even higher, and we can both go out on top."

"I'm not trying to hold you back or stunt your growth, Preacher. If the DEA calls, you should definitely go."

"It's not that I lack confidence in myself, but I still have to pass their selection criteria. Of course I did take some vacation time just to see if that criteria itself is working, or on the beach!"

The chief smiled. "Preacher, you're a scholar and a gentleman. I wish you could take my position!"

"Well, I would, but I'll bet it doesn't come with pralines!"

They both laughed, as Preacher popped the pralines from his hand into his mouth.

"By the way, job well done! I'm glad you weren't hurt." the chief said to Preacher as he shook his hand, then made like he was going to punch him in the stomach, but pulled it."

"Me too, chief."

"Ready to face that media storm?" the chief asked.

"Nope. I'd rather be getting shot at!" Preacher replied.

They both laughed again, as Preacher opened the door to exit the office. Both Preacher and the chief then made their way outside the precinct, where they were immediately greeted with flashbulbs, microphones, and a whole lot of questions.

Chapter Ten

Preacher called Claudine back one last time. It was getting late, so he wanted to find out what course of action she wanted to take. Upon calling he got the answering service, so he called her cell phone.

"Preacher?"

"Hey, Dini."

"I *kinda* figured you wouldn't have this thing wrapped up quick, so I took the kids out. I also made spaghetti and meatballs so you'll have something to eat when you do get in."

"Did you tell the kids what happened?"

There was a brief pause, then Claudine let out a sigh… "The television beat me to it. Your daughter nearly lost her mind when she saw that poor sailor, then the guy with the shotgun get cut down. All she kept screaming was 'Don't let that happen to daddy!' I decided it was best to try and take both of their minds off of it so we went to the movies. Preacher?"

"Yes?"

"You know I understand, and that I don't complain. But you had better stop trying to make me a widow."

"Aw Dini, you know I love you."

"And I love you, but I'm not trying to raise these two kids alone, or with any other man!"

"Trust me. We're gonna live long lives together."

"Okay. I'll remember you said that - while I'm screaming down at you lying in your coffin, trying to climb in it with you!"

"Girl, you crazy!"

"Crazy about you! The movie is about to start. I'll see you later. I love you."

"I love you too, Claudine. Bye."

"Bye."

Preacher's mouth began to water. The thought of chowing down on spaghetti and meatballs had him raring to get home. But home was about to be put off yet again. At that moment, Lieut. Major Merriweather from the Washington DC Metro police came into the precinct. Lieut. Merriweather was a tall, stocky black male. His size was intimidating, but the Lieut. was very reserved and down to earth, only displaying aggressiveness when the situation warranted. He saw Preacher and cheerfully bellowed, "Preach! Caught you on the news. Nice going!"

"Thanks, Major."

"I really came by just to congratulate you in person, but if you're interested, how would you like to come on a raid with us?" the Lieutenant snickered.

Preacher looked at the clock, then shrugged his shoulders. He felt that since he had nothing better to do, he would go on the ride-along.

Chapter Eleven

"Where are we headed?" Preacher asked as the two of them set out in the Lieutenant's patrol car.

"Southeast part of DC, just outside of Prince George's County."

"Ah, yes - the 'Not so *O.K. Corral*'." Preacher said.

Lieut. Merriweather just laughed. "That's why we have to be on top of our game. Can't do much about the drug wars. In fact, there's this one gang out here that's giving us hell. Shutting them down is proving to be a real challenge."

"What do they call themselves?"

"I don't know. I just dubbed them the 'Mayor Marion Barry Marching Band'!"

"Damn, you cold-blooded!" Preacher laughed.

"Actually, it's a crime family. There are so many new Mafia cliques, it's hard to keep track and remember them all!"

"How are you approaching this; hard and fast, or 'Gandhi' style?"

"I've always felt that it's better to knock, than knock down. Don't get me wrong, we're always prepared for violence. But I can say, thanks to the D. E. C., we've been able to avoid the use of flash grenades and scaring innocent people half to death."

"I'm not really familiar with the *D. E. C.,* because we rely on informants more. What is it?"

"It's the Drug Enforcement Computer. A database which flags drug locations under investigation. It also keeps us from stepping on the toes of agencies that may be investigating the same location. Nine out of ten times, we have a successful raid."

"And what about that 10th time?"

"That's when we have to obtain a 'no knock' warrant." Lieut. Merriweather answered.

DC Metropolitan police were already gathered at the location when the Lieutenant and Preacher pulled up. One of the officers with the ranking of Sgt. approached Lieut. Merriweather and Preacher.

"Hi, Lieut. We're all assembled."

"Good." Lieut. Merriweather replied. He surveyed the group of officers amassed, then confidently said, "Okay. Let's score some drugs!" Preacher and the officers chuckled, as they entered the premises. The apartment was in a brownstone, towards the back. A single officer with a battering ram approached first, and stood at the ready. Lieut. Merriweather stood off to the side of the door. He placed his right hand on his firearm, and banged on the door with his left fist as he bellowed out, **"Metropolitan police! Open it up, or we'll open it for you!"**

"All right, all right! Hold on!" came a slightly muffled voice from behind the door.

Though the officer with the battering ram was prepared to bust in, a forcible entry wasn't needed. The sound of locks turning filled the quiet hallway. As the door swung open, Lieut. Merriweather with his right hand still on his firearm pushed his way in first, followed by Preacher, the Sgt., and a little more than a dozen DC officers.

"Back up against the wall! Now turn around!" the lieutenant barked to the man who had opened the door. He then performed a one-handed pat down of the suspect. Upon a satisfactory search which didn't reveal any weapons, the Lieut. then yelled at the suspect, "Sit down over there!", motioning for him to go to the sofa. "You here alone?" the lieutenant asked.

"Yeah, it's just me. But what's this about?" replied the suspect as he sat down. The lieutenant finally removed his hand from his gun, as he reached inside the inner breast pocket of his jacket and pulled out a document.

"We have a warrant to search these premises for illegal drugs. You would be doing yourself a favor by coming clean right now."

"Hey man, there's no drugs up in here." the suspect replied sheepishly.

"That's exactly what I thought you'd say. Sgt., have them rip this place apart like confetti!"

"You all heard the lieutenant; time to clean house!" the sergeant said to the officers behind him.

Immediately and without saying a word, the officers went to work, splitting up into different rooms of the apartment. Some spilled into the bathroom, some into the kitchen, some stayed in the living-dining room area, and the rest fanned out into the four separate bedrooms. As expected, the sound of furniture being pulled up, tossed and broken echoed throughout the apartment. The suspect who opened the door began to protest…

"Come on guys! That's my mother's room!"

"Your mother stays here with you?" Preacher asked.

"Yes! She likes to stay here when she visits me from Georgia!"

"Atlanta?"- Preacher and Lieut. Merriweather exclaimed at the same time.

"No. Not that it's really any of your business, but I am referring to the Republic of Georgia."

"It's more my business than you realize. Let me find out that you are part of one of these Russian crime families, and you're going to wish our healthcare was socialized!" Lieut. Merriweather countered.

"*Politsiya* don't scare me. You are all the same. But I know someone who **cops** fear. That is all I'm going to say."

"Is this supposed to be some sort of threat? Because I'll slap some cuffs on you right now, and you can call that little friend of yours to bail your ass out!" - Lieut. Merriweather fumed.

Just then, the Sgt. who spoke to Lieut. Merriweather interrupted… "Uh, Lieut?"

"Yes, Sgt.?"

"The place is clean."

"Are you sure you left no stone unturned?" Lieut. Merriweather answered. Now another uniformed cop spoke up…

"Lieut., we checked this entire dwelling. We can't find a thing."

Lieut. Merriweather let out an infuriated sigh, then turned to Preacher and said, "You know, I'm missing a steak dinner for this!"

"Elaine cooking again?" Preacher asked.

The lieutenant patted his stomach and replied, "Doesn't she always?" He then said to his officers, "All right men, let's pack up and go home!"

As he and Preacher headed out the apartment first, the suspect who opened the door got off the sofa and yelled out behind them, "Yeah, you do that! And I'll make sure I call my lawyer!"

The lieutenant stopped, turned to look at the suspect, and repeated verbatim, "Yeah, you do that!" before he and Preacher continued to exit.

Back in his patrol car, Lieut. Merriweather turned to Preacher and said, "Man, I apologize. Thought you would get to see a good bust!"

"No problem, Major. I get my fair share! Thanks for inviting me anyway."

"How are those interviews with the DEA coming along?"

"I haven't been called back yet, but I'll keep you informed."

"By the way, you know you still owe me a pool rematch."

"You'll get your rematch! But you know you and Elaine still owe Claudine and me a rematch in Spades!"

"Yeah we spanked *ya*, didn't we? Heh-heh!"

"Heh, heh, heh – don't rub it in!" Preacher huffed.

"Let's make a deal. How about on our next weekend off, we get together. First, you and I will settle the score on our pool game, and then Elaine and I will gently beat you and Claudine in Spades again!"

"Oh, you're that confident you'll beat us again, huh?"

"Yes I am!"

"It's on, *dawg*!"

"Cool!"

Both Lieut. Merriweather and Preacher bumped fists together to seal the pact.

"Let me get on home. It's late, I'm hungry, and I still have to work tomorrow." Preacher said.

"Well, thanks again for accompanying me. I can drop you all the way home if you like."

"I appreciate it, but I need my vehicle."

"You got it."

Major dropped Preacher back at the precinct, where they said their final goodbyes. Preacher then got into his Jeep, hit I-95 North, and drove back home to Laurel, Maryland.

Chapter Twelve

"Look, there's no point in complaining about it now. As long as they didn't find any product, that's all we care about." Seryoga told the person he was speaking with on his cell phone. It was Jaska, the man in DC at the raided safehouse… "And, as long as you didn't get arrested, it's all good… I know they tore the house up. That's why we have the system we have in place. Was 'Nunchaku' with you? Of course. He has his mixed martial arts bullcrap. Why would he have been there? When he gets in, tell him I said, - No. Tell him, Mstislab said to help you clean the place up and get it back in order. We need it ready for the next phase. All right."

Seryoga ended the call, then turned to Mstislab who was having a drink of Vodka straight from the bottle, and enjoying a cigarette…

"You know the cops raided 99 Sydney Terrace."

"As usual," Mstislab nonchalantly replied between puffs. "But of course they didn't find a thing."

"As usual." Seryoga replied.

Mstislab took another drink, wiped the corners of his mouth and took another puff on his cigarette… "Remember when we spoke about New York and Boston for territory?"

"Yes." Seryoga replied.

"After I call this meeting, that's going to develop on a grand scale. There will be other changes as well. The only raid we will be dealing with then is the type that kills roaches! Get on the phone, and tell everyone I want them assembled in Philly. Call my favorite caterer, and order the usual. And Seryoga, one more thing…"

"Yes?"

"Find me two bricks."

"Two bricks?"

"Bricks, cinderblocks, boulders. I don't care if you have to go to Home Depot."

"Um, sure. Two bricks. No problem."

"I'll explain later. And pick up some more vodka on your way back, and a pack of cigarettes."

Seryoga left without saying another word. Mstislab finished the bottle of vodka he was presently drinking, took another puff of his cigarette, and began whistling the melody to a Euro Dance song he heard in a club before.

Chapter Thirteen

'Courtyard' by Marriott hotels provides a picturesque view from its balconies. The ambience is the reason why Mstislab books his functions at that chain. This meeting was no different as Mstislab had Seryoga order his Brigadiers and Pakhans to come to the hotel located near the Philadelphia airport. In one of the conference rooms, one would have thought it was a corporate business function being held. There were deli meats of every type. Cheeses, rolls, chips and dip, fruit, beer, champagne, and of course liquor; tequila, gin, rum, and vodka. When Mstislab threw a party, he spared no expense. But Mstislab's dark side often caused misery for someone else. Mstislab loved to gamble. He frequented Las Vegas, Atlantic City, Tampa, and casinos in Connecticut. While Mstislab gambled as a means to obtain money for his criminal activities, he also did it for recreation, spending money on any random female that would sleep with him. During one particular night in Las Vegas, Mstislab picked up an escort; - a very high-priced escort. They went back to Mstislab's suite, and when they had finished she demanded payment. Mstislab said to her, "That wasn't even worth a complimentary show here."

"Whether you think it was worth it or not, I need to get paid. Do I need to call my driver and bodyguard 'Sven' up here?" she disputed.

"Sweetheart, if that is a threat, you just rolled a '**seven**-out!'"

Mstislab grabbed the escort by her throat, slammed her into the wall, then down on the bed, picked up and slammed her into the wall again. After she lost consciousness, Mstislab grabbed up her purse, checked out of the hotel, boarded a flight returning to DC, and was never prosecuted for that crime. This was a normal routine for Mstislab; just like his meetings which he held at the hotel for important information distribution. With members of his extended organized crime family coming from various places, it was easier to have everyone together in one location, instead of him trying to go see everybody one on one. Though everyone was dressed in civilian clothing, you could tell who was military and who wasn't. As the group mingled with one another, Mstislab and Seryoga walked in. The entire room broke out into applause. Seryoga was carrying a brown paper bag that looked like it had a box inside. He set it at the head of the table where Mstislab would be sitting. It was time for Mstislab to lay out his plan…

"Comrades. It's been a long time since I've used that term. Happy to see all of you made it, and I hope you enjoy my hospitality."

The room broke out into applause again, and Mstislab gestured for everyone to settle down. He then said to Seryoga, "Go pick me up some cigarettes please." After Seryoga left the room, Mstislab got out of his chair, picked up the brown paper bag that Seryoga had been holding, and started to slowly walk around the room. Mstislab began, "It is very hard for me to keep track of all my soldiers and their activities. This is why I hire underbosses. However, if an underboss fails to do their job, then the soldiers will fail as well."

Mstislab reached into the brown paper bag, and pulled out the ear lobe from the driver 'Yuri' that Seryoga had cut off in New York. He then tossed it in the middle of the table, closed the brown paper bag back up, and continued to walk around the room while still addressing the assemblage.

"If you're an underboss and you know who that belongs to, you are doing your job. If you don't know who that piece of ear belongs to…"

Mstislab stopped walking right behind an older Russian man. He leaned forward and said to the man, "Any idea, Stefan?"

"No, Mstislab. I believe all my guys are accounted for." Stefan replied nervously.

"I believe you should go back to bricklaying. Let me help you."

Mstislab took the brown bag and smashed it against Stefan's head so hard; it knocked him out of the chair.

"Mstislab! Have mercy!" Stefan pleaded.

Mstislab tossed the slightly bloody bag of bricks at Stefan on the floor, and said to him, "I do value your association. But if you ever lose control of any of your soldiers again, - my soldiers, there won't be enough cement to bury all of your body parts with. Understood?"

Stefan nodded his head, as Mstislab himself reached out his hand to help him off the floor. After assisting Stefan back into his chair, Mstislab patted him on the shoulder, then made his way back to his own chair, at which point Seryoga returned with his cigarettes. He handed the pack to Mstislab, who gave him a cross look, as he questioned the purchase…

"What the heck is this?"

"It's 'Blu'."

"I don't give a damn about the color."

"No, that's the brand. It's an electronic cigarette. You smoke too much."

"You know the last person who told me I smoked too much, ended up dying."

"How?"

"I killed them. Get me some real cigarettes, and stop caring so much."

Seryoga took back the pack he gave Mstislab and left the conference room again. Mstislab decided to start the meeting and fill Seryoga in on what little he was missing…

"Let's get down to business. Some of you are civilian, some of you are military. I need all of you (glancing over at Stefan again), in order to make this a successful operation. I will tell you what I need, and this is the crew that can make it happen. The disaster industry is growing. There are more shootings across the nation at schools, than animated violence in video games. Now my bread and butter has always been pills, and some of the hard stuff. But we can capitalize off of the fear of America, simply by supplying the demand for guns. With all the new legislation against assault rifles, more and more people are buying weapons before they find out they can't. There are gaping loopholes in this Nation's gun laws, and a lax background check procedure. It's posted all over social media, with people putting their weapons of choice that they bought on their page! But those are the people who can buy guns legally. What about the ones who can't? This is where we come in, particularly since private sales are not under Federal scrutiny. We need guns anyway (gesturing to the room), as they go along with our trade. You just got to have the 'balls' to take people out, like cops if necessary. We have to be ruthless. The catch is distribution. With the help of the Navy, we can distribute more drugs - and weapons through straw purchasing faster and easier by bringing them in to my central distribution hub in New York, then going where we need to go. Yuri had to learn the hard way that slacking off doesn't get any production accomplished. How are things down in Norfolk, anyway, Thomas?" Mstislab directed to a young Caucasian male at the table.

"Security's tight, but I've still got my process together. Of course, deployment would be a problem. What time frame are we talking?"

"Fleet Week. I know it's coming up, which is why this meeting now is so important. By the way, do you or anyone know why Virgil isn't here?"

"Um, he was reassigned. Got orders to San Diego."

Now Mstislab was angry. He pounded his fist on the table and yelled, "WHAT? Why the hell wasn't I told of this sooner? Why didn't he contact me?"

Nobody answered, then Thomas meekly said, "That's not the only set of problems. A lot of guys got reassigned or other, after that bust at 'Little Creek'."

"WHAT BUST? I am going to say this again… WHY, WAS, I, NOT, INFORMED? Know something? If this results in ME going to the 'pokey', I'm going to be poking one of you! Laugh if you want, but I am dead serious!"

Thomas continued, "I heard 'Avaminx' got caught, but I don't think we have to worry about that."

"I, yi, yi!"- Mstislab exclaimed, slapping his forehead as he slumped down in his chair. Then he said in a surprisingly optimistic tone, "You sure he's not gonna talk?"

"Truth be told, even if he does, he's not going to finger anyone. You yourself said that all of us in the upper level have more to lose. 'Avaminx' knows that we'll kill his entire bloodline back in DC if he so much as breathes a syllable about this family." Thomas stated.

Mstislab relaxed and sat upright. He declared, "So now I ask all of you, are you ready to help this family grow? Because once you elevate me to the status of 'Russian Godfather', I will be the most powerful… We will be the most powerful crime family this side of the Kremlin!"

Seryoga returned at that moment with a pack of regular tobacco cigarettes for Mstislab. He immediately took one out and lit it. Though he didn't have a glass of vodka in his hand, he raised it up symbolically for a toast…

"To our family. Consider this 'operation Wooly Mammoth.' And let our success, be the casino that pays for our dreams!"

The room broke out into applause one more time. Mstislab made eye contact with Stefan, and motioned him to pour and bring him a glass of vodka.

Chapter Fourteen

A light mist was just ending. Shamel and Sequoia were coming around the bend on Morningside Drive towards an area dubbed "The Springboard". "The Springboard" was a lookout point down into Morningside Park which was a known drug area. As Shamel and Sequoia neared their destination, dispatch radioed them for their location. Shamel reached for the police radio to respond, only to have Sequoia playfully slap his hand and grab the handset herself…

"Dispatch to BLING unit C-H, what's your location?"

"BLING unit Charlie-Hotel to dispatch, we're 84 at 'the springboard', copy?"

"10-4. BLING units Foxtrot-Delta and Zulu-Oscar are standing by, copy?"

"10-4" Sequoia replied, keying the handset twice. Sequoia then found a parking spot and backed into it. They always tried to avoid double parking when it was feasible, because the unmarked Chevrolet Impala was already a dead giveaway to what they were. Of course the multiple antennas didn't help either…

"So, how's that boyfriend of yours?" Shamel cheerfully asked Sequoia.

"Oh, please! He thinks he's cute now, with his little brokerage job. The guy is a nerd. He doesn't know I'm ready to drop him."

"Aw *Quoia*, give the 'brother' a chance!"

"Listen to you! Backing him up like he's your boy or something." Sequoia replied sarcastically.

"Hey, I'm just saying. You ain't been with 'ol boy but a minute. I mean, did you change the sheets already?"

"What? Excuse you? Humph! Wouldn't you like to know! Of course those sheets could have been (ahem!) christened with someone else's sweat, and blood, and tears, and, uh, other bodily fluid (giggle). But that's not an admission of guilt!"

"Blood? Tears? I don't know what you're talking about."

"Wait a minute. Didn't you tell me before you liked having nails dug into your back?"

"Yeah, and?"

"And that you wanted to get with a woman who could make you cry?"

"So, *whatcha* saying?"

"Shamel, you and I have been through this before. Don't try to play me."

"Well, (yawn) -" Shamel began to stretch, then he got out of the unmarked car and walked around to the driver's side. Sequoia got out also, and came onto the sidewalk with Shamel.

"All I'm saying Sequoia, is that you don't give people a chance."

"Sure I do. I can't help it if I have high standards like you."

"You think my standards are high? Well, they are, but that's beside the point."

"You see who you have on your arm, even though I think you could do better."

"Better than Nova? And what if I tell you that she does make me cry?"

"I would say she must not be deep enough! Every time you thrust, you bang into that pelvic wall and injure yourself!"

Shamel was speechless. He raised his finger, pointed it at Sequoia, retracted it and pointed it again, all the while with his mouth open. Sequoia just laughed…

"See, got nothing to say."

"You know Sequoia… You… Damn! Why am I partners with you?"

"You love me!"

"You're a pain in my ass!"

"You just don't want to admit it, we're good together!"

"Tell you what. I'll become a Muslim, then marry both of you!"

"Oh, hell no! I'm a selfish bitch! I want you all to myself!"

"Okay. Just remember, you said it and I didn't!"

They both laughed. Sequoia took Shamel's arm into hers as they walked over to the ledge. Sequoia was left-handed, so her firearm and all of her utilities were to the left of her body. Dropping Shamel's arm, Sequoia took the police radio out of the left cargo pants pocket and a cell phone out of the hip one, placing them both on top of the ledge. She then took a small pair of binoculars out of her right side pants pocket, opened them, and began scanning the park. Shamel also placed his police radio on top of the ledge and began looking around. Sequoia turned and offered the binoculars to Shamel.

"Wanna peek?"

"Not through some binoculars. Maybe at some cleavage."

"Damn, you disrespectful!" Sequoia playfully ribbed.

"Yeah, but since you're getting ready to cut 'Mr. Right', off, I figured I could be 'Mr. Right now'!"

At that moment, Sequoia's cell phone rang.

"Speaking of the devil, like I really want him calling me anyway." Sequoia said, as she picked up her phone and glanced at the ID displayed on her screen.

"Oh go ahead and answer it. You know he's worried about you." Shamel said.

The phone rang again as Sequoia just held it.

"That's one of his problems. You know what he had the nerve to say to me?" The phone rang again… "He said I should consider being a paralegal or court reporter if I still wanted to be in law enforcement because this job is too dangerous." Sequoia's phone rang again… "Sha, this is coming from a man who was too much of a punk to take me to 'The Bronx Zoo', saying that area up there is too dangerous! What a moron!" Sequoia's cell finally stopped ringing.

"Oh! Was that the same night you called and asked me what I was doing, because you said you were frustrated and needed a drink?"

"Yeah, all because of him!"

"You know he's gonna call back though. Probably thinking you're under siege right now!"

Before Sequoia could respond, her cell phone did ring again. Shamel laughed, and Sequoia replied, "It's not funny! But I'll answer it this time, or his pathetic ass will never stop bugging me! Watch this." Sequoia finally tapped the screen on her phone to take the call. "Hello!"- she answered in a harsh tone of voice, then softened up… "Oh hi baby!.. No, it's kind of noisy here, so I didn't hear my phone ring at first."

Shamel shook his head and laughed. He started making faces at Sequoia, who turned her back to him so she could concentrate on the call… "Oh, I miss you too!.. Say that again?… The 'Kema' stock rose another four points? Wow! Amazing!.. Yes, eventually I will look at that prospectus and let you start a portfolio for me… I know you're concerned about my financial future, and I appreciate it…"

Sequoia then turned around to face Shamel again, and gave him a desperate pleading look of *Will he ever get off this phone?* As she continued to talk, Shamel's own thoughts drifted to that of Nova. He overheard Sequoia say, "This weekend's no good. They told me something about an investigation in *'the Adirondacs', (*The Adirondacs are the mountains in upstate, New York. We all know, most of us will tell a person anything when you don't want to be bothered with them!). I will have mandatory overtime, come Thursday night..."

Then - it was Thursday, and Shamel's birthday. Things couldn't be more perfect. He had worked his day tour, and was off both Friday and the weekend. It was payday. Even though he knew about it, his unit was throwing him a surprise birthday party downtown. Everything was good to go - until Shamel found out that Nova was sick...

"Aw, Nova. I feel bad."

"(Achoo!) – Shamel, you don't feel half as bad as me. I never expected to catch the flu. Now I can't even... (Achoo!) go celebrate your birthday with you."

"(Sigh) Hey, it's okay. I'd better call and let them know I can't make it."

"No, don't do that!"

"But, Nova-"

"Sha, listen to me. It's <u>your birthday.</u> They're expecting you. There's nothing you can do for me. I've already got my medication, soup... I mean, you're being here is nice and all, but it would just make things worse because then I'll feel guilty about you not enjoying your special day. Besides that, I don't want <u>you</u> getting sick!"

"Are you sure?"

Nova pulled Shamel down to her face, and looked in his eyes…"Shamel, if you were going out for any reason other than your birthday, I would have a problem with it. But then again, I don't have the right to make you suffer along with me. Now go, please. Have a drink for us both!"

"All right. I'm going to call and check on you, though."

"That's fine, but I'll be okay."

"I love you."

"I love you too, but don't kiss me! Don't kiss me!"

Nova began to protest as Shamel bent down to kiss her.

"But-" Shamel countered.

"No, no, no! If you want to, on the forehead. My forehead."

Shamel then planted a kiss on Nova's forehead, which was *hotter than a pot of boiling water on an open flame*. He hugged her and said, "Take care, feel better." as he headed out of her apartment.

Shamel opted for mass transit, since he knew he would be drinking. The bus arrived and Shamel boarded, flashing his shield for a courtesy ride. Taking a seat near the rear door, Shamel closed his eyes and dozed off. He was in good spirits, and knew the party would only enhance his mood. After the bus arrived at its final destination, Shamel exited and began the trek to the bar. He grew giddy the closer he got. A few people who Shamel recognized were standing outside the bar, smoking. As soon as one of them noticed Shamel, they all waved to him, then quickly disappeared inside. Shamel chuckled as he got right up to the door. He went inside, and was immediately greeted with, "Surprise! Happy birthday, Shamel!" from the entire bar. Sequoia ran up and gave him a kiss on the cheek, and a hug. Someone handed him a beer, while someone else motioned for the bar to quiet down. Angel then approached Shamel and began speaking…

"Shamel, on behalf of the NYPD, we toast you on being another year older. But you can't keep stealing that black market 'Cialis' out of the evidence locker!"

The entire bar responded with "Whoa!" while Shamel stood there in embarrassed modesty. This wasn't a party - it was a roast! Shamel caught it from his entire unit. He even caught a ribbing from members of other units he knew. Seemed like everybody showed up; the Organized Crime Control Bureau, Highway and Mounted patrols, Major Case Squad, Emergency Service Unit… Shamel took it all in stride, for there was nothing like being shown love!

As the party was winding down, Shamel felt very tipsy from his alcohol consumption. He still had his faculties about him, but now was the time to act silly…

"We had to put them in their place, because they were out of line!" - Detective-Sgt. Degrella was telling the table Shamel was seated at with other members of his unit. She was a very pretty, full figured older black woman who orientated all detectives new to B.L.I.N.G.

"So, Shamel, are you going to tell the story or should I?"

"Um, well-"

She cut Shamel off by assertively grabbing his head, and resting it on her ample bosom. She then began to gently stroke his head as Shamel helplessly but willingly laid there, let out a sigh, closed his eyes and smiled.

"Anyway," she continued; "Shamel hadn't been with this unit even 90 days, and already was getting into trouble! We were on a routine buy and bust operation. In fact, all we were supposed to do was make a sale and walk away. Shamel posed as the buyer, while Detective Shepherd and I provided surveillance to make sure things went smoothly. But as soon as Shamel completed the transaction with the dealer, this car came out of nowhere, and two white males with guns jumped out. Mind you, we're watching the whole thing unfold. They had no emergency lights on their vehicle and no badges displayed, so at first we thought it was a surprise attack. Then I heard one of them yell 'Freeze!' The dealer took off and had one of these guys chase after him, while Shamel started backing up."

"Yeah, I was trying to get my badge out." Shamel said.

"Hush, I'm telling the story!" Detective-Sgt. Degrella said to Shamel. "So anyway, before Shamel could really react, the other guy tackles him! He rolled Shamel over, puts his knee into the back of his neck, and starts cursing him out." Pausing to take a breath, Detective-Sgt.Degrella took another sip of her drink, then continued… "At this point, we figure out they're cops from another unit. Just so happened, as Detective Shepherd and I began approaching them, the guy who tackled Shamel takes his badge out from under his shirt, and is preparing to put cuffs on him. So we walk up with our shields hanging from around our necks, and I said to the guy, 'Excuse me, that's a fellow officer you just took down.' He had this surprised look on his face, and then he gets up and lets Shamel up as well. After he holsters his weapon, he says to Shamel, 'No hard feelings, dude.' (Giggling) - and Shamel says to him, 'Nah, no hard feelings - just a hard fist!' after which he decked him right in the face!"

Everyone around the table started laughing. Shamel raised his head which she finally let go of and retorted, "You know I caught a week's suspension behind that with no pay!"

"True, but I found out that both of those cops got suspended without pay for 30 days, and were transferred to less than desirable units! Ah, my sources at One Police Plaza!" Detective-Sgt. Degrella finished.

"Heck, Sha's more than made up for that week, with all the mandatory overtime we do!" Sequoia said.

"Well, that's it for me. Have to be in court in the morning. Shamel, happy birthday again!" Detective-Sgt. Degrella said as she rose out her seat. Giving Shamel a hug and a light peck on the lips, she then said to Sequoia, "Sequoia, you keep him out of trouble. We certainly don't want him ending up in traffic enforcement!"

"I know. Some people have mighty long weekends till Monday!" Sequoia joked.

"Whatever!" Shamel replied.

"I'm gone. Take care."

"Bye." Shamel said to Detective-Sgt. Degrella.

After she left, Viper said, "This party was all right, especially the catered sandwiches. Did you guys try the ham?"

Shamel then said, "Speaking of ham, I got a joke for *ya*!"

"Oh lord; here goes the black 'Jay Leno'! Sequoia jeered.

"Oh come on, it's funny! You guys ready?"

"Yeah, yeah, sure…" - the entire table responded.

Shamel took a drink of his beer, then began… "What do you call a pig on crack?" Everyone just looked at each other, then Shamel answered, "Sizzle-lean!" That joke did earn Shamel a few laughs, so feeling encouraged, he continued… "Is a pig in charge, considered to be Boss Hog? Is a pig in bondage, hog-tied? What's the difference between a pig in a blanket and a pig under a blanket?"

"More oinking when you're 'boinking'?" Angel asked.

"Ill, that's disgusting!" Sequoia countered.

"Well, Angel's close. The answer is, you don't sleep with pigs <u>in</u> a blanket!" Shamel said.

"Okay, I think you and your pig jokes need to wallow on home now." Sequoia challenged.

"One more. Where do pigs on drugs go for rehab?" Everyone just looked at Shamel. Then with a big grin, he said, "De - Chops! Piggy Detox!"

"All right, I've heard enough! You're drunk!" Sequoia rebuked.

Shamel turned to Sequoia and said, "I gotta admit, I'm toasted! Don't know how much longer I'm going to be *chillin* here myself."

"Well it's not like you have to work in the morning. Hang out, I'll take you home."

"Would ya, *pardtner*?"

"Sure, p*ardtner*!" Sequoia giggled.

"Well then, um, I have a favor to ask."

"Okay?" Sequoia questioned.

"Sequoia, would you…"

"Yes?"

"Would you…"

"*Yeaaa?..*"

Now the entire table was looking at Shamel inquisitively. Shamel finished his beer, then said,

"Would you – take off your bra?"

Sequoia's mouth dropped open, as the rest of the table burst out into laughter.

"Shamel, I don't believe you! Hell no! I ain't taking off my bra!"

"Yeah but the bar-"

"I know all about the taking off of the bra, putting it with the rest of them behind the bar and trying to guess how many are there… - No! I'm not doing it! Sorry!"

"Well, would you at least dance with me at the bar?" Shamel pleaded.

"I'm not taking off my bra." Sequoia replied again.

Both of them got up and made their way over to the bar where at the encouragement of the bartenders and other patrons, they both got up on the bar counter itself. One of the bartenders handed Shamel a nearly empty bottle of Bacardi Hurricane, which Shamel put to his mouth and finished downing. Music from the jukebox was blaring Pink Floyd's "Empty Spaces". Shamel and Sequoia began dancing, with Sequoia gyrating her hips into Shamel's groin. She tapped her butt with her left hand twice as Shamel steadied himself with both hands on her back. All this occurred while Pink Floyd belted out these lyrics to the song:

"Oooh, I need a dirty woman… Oooh, I need a dirty girl…"

The whooping and yelling went on until the bartenders announced, "Last call for alcohol!" As the bar cleared out and everyone was saying goodbye, Sequoia offered for Shamel to stay the night at her apartment. She hoped Shamel would take up the offer, being as she was tired and didn't live far from the bar anyway. Sequoia was a bit under the influence of alcohol herself, while Shamel was intoxicated…

"I can call a cab, *Quoia*."

"Now why do that, so he can take advantage and overcharge you for a trip uptown? Boy, you better come over to this apartment and sleep it off!"

Shamel quit protesting. Sequoia helped him into her car, and off they went. Upon arriving at her building, Sequoia assisted Shamel out of the car, and helped him drag himself up to her apartment. Once inside, Sequoia walked Shamel over to the sofa…

"Ok, Sha, here you go. Man, are you heavy!"

"I don't weigh that much. Must be my bladder!"

"Well I'm telling you now. Pee on my sofa, and it's *gonna be one*!" Sequoia took off Shamel's shoes and placed his feet on the sofa. "Let me get you a blanket."

"O-k, blank… cool."

Shamel was becoming incoherent. Sequoia went to her linen closet, took a blanket out and brought it back to Shamel. Unfolding it, she draped it over his body leaving his head exposed.

"Hey, Quoia?"

"Yes?"

"Thank. Thanks – you."

Shamel fell asleep just that quick. Sequoia smiled and quietly replied, "You're welcome, partner." Sequoia then went to the bathroom to wash up, and went to bed - where she was immediately set upon by 'the Sandman' herself.

Shamel awoke in the morning to the aroma of bacon and eggs. Although Sequoia had to go to work, she left Shamel breakfast and a note on the coffee table that read, "Hope your hangover isn't too bad. Just make sure you raise my toilet seat when you pee! *Luv* Sequoia."

Shamel ate, washed his dishes, and then called Nova to check on her. Nova was a bit livid at learning that Shamel spent the night someplace other than home…

"But Nova, all I did was go to sleep! Honest!.. Oh come on, Nova. I know you're still not feeling well. But if I was gonna cheat, why would I call you from another woman's place? Seriously, Sequoia and I are just coworkers and friends, you know that. I was piss drunk last night, - well, everybody was, and couldn't make it back to Harlem!.. Yeah, I'm still off today. I'm off this whole weekend remember?.. Of course I'm going to come by and see you. In fact, I'll spend the entire day with you. You know, make you some more soup, cuddle up and try to help you sweat that flu out of your body!.. I love you too, see you soon… Huh? What's that about Mars? Mars…"

"EARTH TO MARS!" - Sequoia hollered at Shamel. She was done with her phone conversation, and trying to get Shamel's attention while he was still daydreaming. Startled, Shamel tried to play it off, and began scratching his back…

"Damn! Can't get that itch for nothing."

"You ain't slick, boy. Popped into one of your little worlds again, *didn'tcha*?" Sequoia confronted. "We've been partners for too long. I know you better than you know yourself!" Shamel just made a face. "Anyway, I'm sure you want to see this." Sequoia handed Shamel the binoculars. “Look North. Black jacket, black denim and work boots.”

Shamel looked through the binoculars and saw what Sequoia was referring to. It was a drug dealer. Though business didn’t seem too brisk for him, Shamel observed a sale being conducted. It was time to *spring* into action…

“Okay, we’ll let the buyer go. I want this guy, so I’ll go down and secure him.”

“Want me to come with you?” Sequoia asked.

“No. Stay here just in case he runs. You can back me up faster than the other units.”

“Gotcha, *Kojack*. Be careful.”

Shamel turned and pointed both of his index fingers at Sequoia, then said, “Who loves ya, baby?” before continuing on down into the park. As he approached the dealer, his gait was neither fast nor slow. In fact, Shamel tried to be as nonchalant as possible, but it didn’t work. Maybe the dealer knew what the ‘color of the day’ was. Maybe his instincts were very perceptive. Maybe he simply didn’t trust an unfamiliar husky black male coming in his direction. In any case, the dealer started to walk away. Shamel yelled out, "Stop!", but the dealer ignored the command and went into a sprint. The chase was on.

Chapter Fifteen

"You don't catch hell, because you're a Mason or an Elk. You don't catch hell, because you're a Democrat or a Republican, and you sure don't catch hell because you're an American – Cause if you were an American, you wouldn't catch no hell! You catch hell – Because you're a Black Man!" - **Malcolm X**

Shamel took off after the dealer with lightning speed. Meanwhile, Sequoia who observed the drama unfold jumped back into the unmarked police cruiser. With emergency lights flashing and siren wailing, she took off down Morningside Drive with the intent of assisting Shamel in apprehending the suspect. The drug suspect had no intention of being caught. He stopped short, spun around rapidly, and began firing off rounds from a 9mm handgun. Shamel dove for cover and immediately assumed the combat position. Fortunately, none of the rounds struck Shamel. Bullets flew wildly as the dealer recklessly and callously aimed from side to side in an attempt to hit him. A lot of chaos ensued, but luckily the rain had kept most people out of the park. However, the few people who were there posed a very big risk. Everyone tried to run for cover when the shooting began. A couple that was picnicking cowered behind a tree. A mother with her infant child in a stroller snatched the baby out of it and ran as fast as she could out of the park. Other people were either running or laying on the ground, unsure what to do. Shamel took a quick scene survey - and displayed incredible restraint. Assessing that too many lives were at risk, he did not return fire. He waited until the dealer resumed running, then took off after him again. Unfortunately, Shamel didn't see a low hanging branch from a tree and ran dead smack into it, resulting in a gash above his left eye. It stunned him for a moment, but he shook it off and kept after the dealer. The dealer had a slight bit of distance on Shamel, and figured he could get rid of Shamel altogether by heading into the subway. However, his escape plan didn't work out the way he wanted. He hopped the turnstile, but missed a local downtown train that just pulled out. So he did the unthinkable, and jumped onto the tracks in a bid to try to escape back outside. Express 'A' and 'D' trains traveling in both directions narrowly miss him as he precariously stepped over the third rails crossing over to the other platform. Shamel made it down to the station and witnessed the dealer crossing the tracks. At first, Shamel was going to do the same, then he decided a better strategy was to go back up to the street. As Shamel scrambled back up the stairs, the dealer was climbing onto the platform on the other side. Shamel made it back up to street level, and began to wildly dodge traffic trying to cross over. A lot of vehicles came to a screeching halt as Shamel bobbed and weaved to avoid being hit, but he wasn't about to let the dealer get away under any circumstances. By now, the dealer had made it up the stairs of the other platform himself as Shamel predicted. He came out of the station and was about to run across the street back to the park when Sequoia pulled up in the cruiser, blocking his path. She jumped out with her weapon drawn and yelled, "Freeze!" That's when the dealer made a critical error. He was literally face-to-face with Sequoia when he tried to draw his weapon again (as he wasn't smart enough to ditch it during the chase!). In one swoop motion – and with only one hand free, Sequoia grabbed and wrenched his arm, forcing him to drop his gun. She then delivered a powerful well-placed kick to the dealer's solar plexus, and took him down hard! Sequoia stepped behind him, put her knee in the back of his neck and pinned his arm behind him.

"You're under arrest! Move and I'll blow your head off!" Sequoia yelled eagerly but calmly.

Shamel was a bit out of breath when he caught up to Sequoia. Taking care not to contaminate the handle of the 9mm with his own fingerprints, Shamel picked up the dealer's weapon by the barrel and after switching it from 'fire' to 'safe', placed the weapon in the cargo pocket of his pants for the time being. Sequoia continued the arrest by placing handcuffs on the dealer.

"Nice work partner! You okay?" Shamel gasped.

“I’m fine. Are you okay? Looks like you caught a serious ‘speed knot’! Sequoia replied.

“Yeah, I’m good. Just wanted to catch this scumbag!”

The dealer was squirming a bit, as Sequoia still had her knee in the back of his neck…

“Yo, I can’t breathe!” the dealer exclaimed.

Shamel looked down at him and replied, “That’s interesting. If you couldn’t breathe, you wouldn’t be able to talk!” After the dealer was cuffed, Shamel took over. He assertively picked the dealer up off the ground, slammed him onto the left fender of the police cruiser and said, “You have the right to remain silent. If you give up this right – I’ll be so *got-damn* happy!”

Upon that, he strong-armed the dealer into the back seat of the police cruiser. Things had occurred and unfolded so quickly – yet, it was over. The other two units on standby comprised of Viper and Lavender and detectives Zhao and O’Brannon made their way down to Adam Clayton Powell Boulevard and 135th St. in front of the subway station to assist. Shamel waived and signaled to them that everything was under control. Sequoia got on the police radio to request an ambulance for Shamel, and a tour supervisor for the shooting investigation. Fortunately, Shamel was the only one mildly injured. Except for a shattered car window on the street from a spent shell, no other casualties were produced. An excited crowd of onlookers began to form, and traffic began to back up with rubberneckers.

Shamel sat on the hood of the police cruiser to wait for the ambulance, while the other detectives in the two back up units began to both render crowd control and direct traffic.

Chapter Sixteen

FDNY-EMS arrived very quickly. The crowd was fairly large-scale but some marked blue and white units as well as the NYPD traffic division had arrived on the scene to assist. The tour supervisor ordered the dealer to be placed in a blue and white patrol car for his trip to the hospital to be medically cleared before going to arraignment. Shamel was now sitting on the floor of the back of the ambulance being treated for the laceration he sustained during the chase. By chance, he knew the medics who arrived, so they took extra liberty in treating him…

"I'd suture you up right here if I could!" the first paramedic said to Shamel, while the second was writing up the ambulance call report.

"I appreciate it Tamra, but I need some aspirin. This thing 'smarts'!" Shamel replied.

"Thought you were 'Tonka' tough!" Sequoia said.

"I am, but tree branches and skin don't mix!" Shamel replied.

"Don't worry baby, I'll fix you up and take good care of you!" Tamra said.

"Watch that, before I have to get his girlfriend on you!" Sequoia said, pretending to be serious.

"*I am* his girlfriend!" Tamra chuckled, giving Shamel a one-arm hug.

"Which facility do you want to go to, Sha?" the second paramedic asked.

"Take me to Columbia-Presbyterian, since that perp is going to Harlem Hospital."

"You got it. Just watch your head going inside the 'bus'." the second paramedic said.

He walked around to the driver's side of the ambulance, while Shamel and the first paramedic climbed into the back. Sequoia went to the police cruiser to follow behind them for the trip to the hospital. Both vehicles drove at a quick yet cautious pace with emergency lights flashing, and intermittent use of their sirens. The second paramedic had called ahead, so medical staff in the ER at Columbia

Presbyterian was on standby awaiting Shamel's arrival to expedite his treatment and release

Chapter Seventeen

The tour supervisor dropped by the ER to check up on Shamel, who was being discharged. He spoke with Shamel briefly, and then walked away. At that moment, Sequoia knocked on the door of the exam room, and popped her head inside...

"So, how's my partner in anti-crime?" she mused.

Shamel put on a phony attitude... "They're letting me go! No bland food tonight! (Sniff!)"

"Well, at least you got some time off!"

"Yeah! Tour supervisor said I could take a week and more if needed. I just have to contact the nypd physician for clearance."

"Is the tour supervisor still around?"

"I think so. Check by the vending machines. He told me he was going to grab a cup of coffee."

Sequoia flashed a broad smile... "Be right back!" she quickly uttered, and dashed off toward the vending machine area.

As Shamel continued getting dressed, the nurse came into the room...

"Here's some Tylenol, detective. Did you receive your discharge instructions?"

"Yes, Nurse."

"You're all set then. Take care and good luck."

"Thank you."

Shamel swallowed down the pills, and had just finished putting his shirt back on when Sequoia reentered the room. She was sulking, and didn't look cheery one bit…

"Ill! What's up with that sour-puss? Looking like someone *done* stole your birthday cake! Just a minute ago, you were as happy as a **chicken** on Thanksgiving day!"

"Well…" Sequoia began. "I thought I could get off too. But the supervisor said since **I** wasn't actually injured and they were short staffed, – hey, you know the deal!"

"Sorry they wouldn't let you go as well." Shamel said.

"It doesn't matter. What's important is that you're okay. So, got any plans for your sudden vacation?"

"Yeah. I need to catch up with some judges. Judge Mathis, Judge Joe Brown, Judge Judy…"

"Fool!" - Sequoia laughed. Shamel opened his arms, and Sequoia willingly embraced him.

"Whatever you do, be safe, and think about me from time to time!" Sequoia chimed.

"Or as they say, don't do anything I wouldn't do, right?" Shamel replied.

Shamel then hopped off the exam table, and exited to the waiting room with Sequoia where Viper, Lavender, Zhao and O'Brannon were waiting for them…

"How do you feel, Sha?" Viper asked.

"Hungry! We missed lunch." Shamel replied.

"Then let's go get some chow; - Chinese food!" Detective Zhao suggested.

All six of them filed back out to their unmarked patrol cars, and drove to Chinatown for a bite to eat, before returning to the precinct.

Chapter Eighteen

A shoe here. Garment bags and suitcases of clothing there. Marked boxes lined and stacked all about the apartment. It was moving day for Nova. She and Shamel along with a handful of Shamel's coworkers from the precinct had toiled since early morning to get her moved into Shamel's place. Now they were both relaxing and getting settled. Nova had already showered, and was preparing to update her resume. She came out of the bathroom wearing a robe, and had a towel wrapped around her head. Shamel was in his underwear, preparing to enter the shower. As they were passing each other in the hallway, they paused to kiss. Shamel then playfully slapped Nova on her butt. She emitted a gleeful shriek and muttered an audible "Fresh!" as he went into the bathroom, and she went to sit down at the computer. Nova logged into the Internet radio station on Shamel's computer to listen to music as she worked. The genre was Latin Jazz; the artist was 'Michel Camilo', and the track was 'Poinciana'. Shamel turned on the shower. Nova turned on her own laptop. Michel Camilo played. Shamel stepped in under the shower head. Nova inserted her USB into the USB port. Michele Camilo played on. Shamel adjusted the water temperature. Nova scrolled to Microsoft Word. Michele Camilo played on. Shamel picked up the soap and his face cloth. Nova clicked on "file", "open", and opened her resume Word document. Michele Camilo played on. Shamel scrubbed. Nova adjusted her font sizes. Michele Camilo played on. Shamel washed his hair. Nova's finger slipped off the Shift key and hit the Enter key. Michele Camilo played on. Shamel rinsed off. Nova pressed Ctrl + Z. Michele Camilo played on. Shamel dried off, and donned a clean pair of boxer shorts. Nova clicked the spell check icon. Michele Camilo played on. Shamel brushed his teeth. Nova clicked the "Save" icon. Michele Camilo played on. Shamel flexed in front of the mirror and growled. Nova was revising her "objective" and growling. Michele Camilo was still playing. The telephone rang...

"Nova! Answer that please." Shamel yelled out.

"Ooh, Sha! I'm in the middle of a thought!" Nova yelled back.

Shamel made a face at her as he walked out into the living room and said, "I'll give you something to be in the middle of!"

"*Perv*!" Nova muttered.

Shamel looked at the caller ID and chuckled. It was Preacher. By now the phone was on its fourth ring but Shamel picked it up…

"Hey, Preach!" – And Michele Camilo was done…

"Shamel! Sorry I'm just now getting back to you. Glad you're okay."

"Yeah, I'm fine, though I've probably got some extra grey hairs from that!"

"Did you go to the arraignment?"

"Hell yeah! Mom, Venice, and Deneen came too."

"That's good! Our sisters are a little *tight* with me right now, because they feel I should have made my way up to New York for moral support, considering my own shootout episode weeks back."

"It's ok. It's not like I actually took a bullet, though it felt like it!"

"I know, but you know that 'baby breath' and 'ne-ne' ain't trying to hear that."

"Were you on three-way with them?"

"Uh-huh. Venice was telling me to hop on 'Amtrak' and come through. I explained to her that I got the message from Nova, and spoke to Mom who also told me you weren't hurt bad. If it were a life and death situation, I would do what I have to do."

"No doubt. Did you explain to them that you also cannot teleport?"

"(Cackle) Yes. Then I called you, but it went to your voice mail."

"I probably had my phone on silent then. We made Night Court and it was packed."

"What did the court say?"

"They indicted him on drug and weapons possession, as well as two counts of attempted murder of a law enforcer and reckless endangerment. And the best part (chuckle), he was denied bail! Man, when

Sequoia and I got outside the courthouse, we started dancing around like two little kids. People looked at us like we were crazy, or had just been released from lockup ourselves!"

"That's what's up! How's Sequoia anyway?"

"She's fine, just a little *pissy* because the department wouldn't give her anytime off as well."

"She wasn't in the line of fire, huh?"

"You guessed it!"

Claudine had just brought Preacher a glass of cranberry juice. She decided to butt in at that moment, and took Preacher's phone out of his hand…

"Hey, Shamel!"

"Hi, Claudine!"

"You and your brother seem to have a penchant for gunfights nowadays."

"It's not our fault, Claudine!" Shamel pleaded.

At that moment, Nova decided to join the conversation… "Ooh! That's Claudine? I want to talk to her!"

Shamel put the phone on speaker, so they could both talk at once.

"Hey, Claudine!"

"Hi, Nova! Shamel better be treating you right!"

"Well you know we just moved in together. I guess time will tell."

"Habits, habits. You have to be able to tolerate a person's habits." Shamel interjected.

"That's so true. I still can't get used to this one snoring!" Claudine replied.

"Hell woman, you snore too! And that is not a habit! " Preacher snapped.

"It is if you do it every night! Also, I don't snore as loud as you, 'Toro'!"

"Toro?"

"Yes, as in lawn mower! Rrrrr!"

Shamel and Nova fell out laughing, while Preacher and Claudine continued fussing at each other for a brief moment…

"Let me get back to what I was doing, before this one decides to cuff me in the bedroom!" Claudine said.

"Ah, *ya* into that freaky stuff, huh?" Shamel snickered.

"I didn't say it had anything to do with sex. I just said he was going to cuff me in the bedroom!"

"Yeah, get you out of my hair for a while!" Preacher said.

"See? The male version of 'Kathy Bates' from 'Misery'! Anyway, great talking to you, Nova and Shamel. Will we see you guys soon?"

"I was just going to speak to them about that." Preacher said.

"Okay! Speak to you soon then! Bye!" Claudine finished.

"Bye, Claudine!" - Nova and Shamel both replied.

Claudine kissed Preacher on the lips and handed his phone back to him, then walked away. Preacher resumed speaking to Shamel and Nova… "You know Sha, the kids miss you. It would be nice if you two could come down for little while especially since I'm on vacation."

"So early?" Shamel asked.

"Let me cut to the chase. I was anticipating another round of interviews with the DEA, but they haven't called. I'm still taking my vacation though!"

"I hear that! Well, Nova and I will gladly come on down."

"You know you're always welcome. Okay, let me go cuff my wife now!"

"You better leave her alone!" Nova laughed.

"You know I got jokes! Listen, you two take care. I will see you soon!" Preacher replied.

"That you will bro! Love you!" Shamel said.

"Love you, Preacher!" Nova said also.

"Love you guys too. Bye."

"Bye!"- Shamel and Nova both replied as Shamel pressed the speaker phone off.

"Yaaa, we get to get out of the city! I'm so excited!" Nova exclaimed.

"Me too! Plus it will be good to bond with-"

"My future in-laws?" Nova enthusiastically butted in.

"Uh, can we get past the 'honeymoon phase', before a real Honeymoon?" Shamel chided.

"My bad, I thought we were halfway there!" Nova answered.

"I can't wait to be halfway to Maryland! We haven't had a road trip in a while. I need to calm my nerves!" Shamel bemoaned.

"Oh you big baby, I'll help you calm your nerves." Nova cooed.

Shamel jokingly began to stutter...

"I (sniff!), I, j, j-just ww-went through a tra – tra – traumatic experience. Have you no sympathy?"

"Of course I do. I have sympathy, empathy, and telepathy (giggle)."

"Telepathy, huh? Hmm. So, what am I thinking right now?" Shamel valiantly asked.

"That you want to levitate me to passion!" Nova said softly.

They both giggled, then kissed. Nova squealed with delight as Shamel picked her up and carried her into the bedroom. They embraced in a passionate kiss, as

Shamel gently placed her on the bed. Lying next to her on her right side, they continued kissing as Shamel undid her robe. Nova sat up and took the robe completely off, as well as the towel from her head. One thing about Nova; she had the type of body that would make a man drool. Standing at 5'9", her 40 DD breasts along with her 38 inch hips and caramel/bronze complexion definitely gave Shamel the *high-rise* that she didn't mind climbing! Nova began to pull down Shamel's boxer shorts which he helped take off. His well-endowed *chocolate* shaft was already rock hard. Resuming their kissing, Shamel began to gently fondle Nova's right breast, taking effort to manipulate and tease her hard nipple with his fingers. Shamel then started kissing Nova on her neck, and gently caressed both of her breasts. Nova responded with soft moans of delight. Finally, Shamel's tongue made it to the nipples. First he licked each nipple, applying gentle pressure with each stroke. He gently bit and held the right nipple between his teeth, before swallowing and sucking on as much of her breast as he could. Shamel did this without using his hands. He then repeated the same for the left nipple and breast, adjusting his suction according to the intensity of Nova's sighs; if she sighed softly, he increased pressure. If she sighed loudly - - he increased pressure till she arched her back.

"Ummm, stop teasing me." Nova pleadingly sighed.

Shamel just snickered. Things were about to get intense. Real intense. Real steamy.

Nova playfully pushed Shamel down, and began to lick his nipples. She slid her hand down to his penis and began stroking it, caressing his balls as well. But then Shamel playfully pushed Nova back down, asserting, "I'm in charge here." as sensually as he could.

"*S'cuse* me, you big-dick mother-fucker! Show me whatcha got!" Nova dared.

Upon that, Shamel resumed licking Nova's nipples and breasts, when his left hand made its way down to her vagina. First, Shamel played with Nova's soft pubic hairs, managing to curl a few strands around his pinky finger. He then began to gently rub the outer lips, getting them extra moist from her natural lubrication. Finally, Shamel's slipped two of his fingers inside of her. He honed in on the clitoris, and began to gently tweak and rub it. The rubbing transformed to quick little flicks, with Shamel's finger rapidly jiggling the sensitive organ, intermittently applying pressure as well. Nova's breathing slowed and deepened. She tried to look at Shamel, but her eyes were rolling in her head. At last she gave up, closed them, and began making audible moans of pleasure. Shamel paused to give Nova a kiss on her lips. He pressed his hard penis against her left thigh, and rubbed his hips up and down. Shamel then parted Nova's thighs open and said to her, "Bye-for now." as he rose up and slid down till his mouth was at her *pond of pleasure*. Nova was so wet already; Shamel's tongue was doing laps, as he lapped up the sweet love juice that her 'sugar walls' were producing…

"Ohhh, damn! Sha, don't stop"…

Nova gasped as Shamel fiercely licked her entire vaginal orifice. He gave her clit extra attention, both gently biting and sucking the flesh like it was a piece of peppermint candy. Nova took her hands and held Shamel's head down - - just the way he liked it! Shamel took his hands and clasped hers. Through a muffled voice (well, what else did you expect?) he said to Nova,

"I wanna taste it. Let it go in my mouth."

"Ohh, baby, don't stop!" Nova begged.

Shamel continued for about a minute, then he felt Nova's body tense up. Nova's breathing quickened, and her grip on Shamel's head grew tighter.

"Oh damn, I'm about to *cum*, Sha! I'm going to *cum*!" – Nova eked out in a high pitched voice. Shamel grabbed Nova's hips, and forced his face deep into her love zone. A few final, deliberate, powerful strokes of his tongue, and Nova let out an "Ohhhhhh!" along with her orgasm. Shamel continued to furiously lick all around; to the point where Nova had to plead for him to stop as she pushed his head away and allowed her body to relax. Shamel lovingly gazed up at Nova who lovingly gazed back at him. He then went to the night table drawer, took out a small travel size bottle of mouthwash and had a swallow, after which he kissed Nova on her lips again. Nova gently caressed Shamel's still erect penis, then leaned forward and popped the tip into her mouth. She let it slide back out, flicked her tongue over the slit, then swallowed it again as she fondled Shamel's *nuts,* causing him to moan with delight. Motioning for Shamel to lie down, Nova slowly continued to engulf his entire cock in her mouth. Shamel softly called out Nova's name, as she leisurely performed oral sex on him. Leaning over, Shamel stroked her head, and ran the tips of his fingernails up and down her back. Nova moved her mouth from Shamel's penis to his balls, gently licking and sucking on them, just like he did to her clit. But after about a minute of that, Shamel stopped her.

"Hey, I'm not done!" Nova whined.

"Oh yes you are! I want you, now."

Shamel repositioned his body, so the two of them were face to face again with Nova on the bottom. They interlocked their fingers as they kissed, intertwining their tongues. Shamel motioned for Nova to roll over.

He caressed her ass, as he ran his tongue from the top of her ear, inside her ear, down her neck to her shoulder blades, and down her spine. Now Shamel was positioned directly behind Nova. He kissed both of her butt cheeks, then gave them a firm slap.

"Ooh!" Nova responded. In a seductive show of readiness, Nova made her butt cheeks clap together.

"You 'bout to really get spanked now!" Shamel boldly announced.

"Mmm, yeah. Bring it on baby!" Nova hummed.

Shamel parted Nova's cheeks as she assumed the doggie position. He slipped inside of her very effortlessly, and began to pump away, with his balls slapping her ass on every stroke.

"Oh yeah! Mmmm!" Nova murmured.

"Ah, yeah. Pussy's nice and deep!" Shamel grunted.

"Just for you, baby!" - Nova gasped as she took Shamel's thumping.

He grabbed Nova's hair will one hand, and braced the other on her hip as the pumping intensified. Then, Shamel slowed, and finally pulled out. He rolled Nova over. As she willingly spread her thighs wide open to receive him, he injected his *love syringe* into her subcutaneous juicy folds. Shamel braced himself with his arms spread about her midsection, as he began to thrust in and out, like a well-oiled piston. He changed his rhythm, and grabbed one of her butt cheeks as he began to grind his hips, before switching back to the thrusts. They kissed. They humped. They moaned. They pumped. Shamel felt his body grow tense, as he neared the scream of passion. His breathing deepened, and his grip tightened just a bit. Nova responded by gripping Shamel tight as well…

"I'm getting close girl!" Shamel gasped.

"Take me with you! I'm so close too! Ready to cum again!" Nova blurted out.

Their lovemaking intensified. Beads of sweat dripped from Shamel's forehead onto Nova's chest.

"Are you close?" Shamel asked.

"Yes, baby!" Nova replied.

"Are you close?" Shamel asked again.

"I'm right there! Oh, Sha, I'm about to cum!"

"Me too! Right there! Cum with me!"

"Yes!"

"Cum WITH ME!"

"YES!"

"OH, NOVA! NOVA! I'M - AHHHH!"

"ME TOO-OHHHH!"

Their legs interlocked tighter and their grip on each other strengthened, as Shamel and Nova climaxed together. Shamel felt Nova's vaginal muscles tighten, while she felt Shamel's 10 inches of *dickmeat* pulse, throb, and unload deep inside her *jizz tunnel*. Shamel and Nova kissed, sighing "I love you." to each other in between, as the tension in their bodies slowly dispersed. Shamel stayed mounted for about a minute afterwards. Ever so gingerly, he slowly pulled out of Nova, and lay next to her, caressing her face as they continued kissing, flicking their tongues and rubbing their noses together. Shamel closed his eyes, as his body began to totally relax. Their kissing slowed, but Nova kept on giving Shamel light pecks on his lips, and observed him as he dozed off. She watched how he breathed, smiling at him the entire time. After about 20 minutes had passed, Nova tried to wake him…

"Sha?" Nova spoke softly.

No response. Flatline. Shamel was *dead*.

"Shamel?" Nova spoke a bit louder now.

A sign of life. Shamel stirred. He still wasn't resurrected yet though…

"Shamel?" Nova said again, this time gently nudging him. Alas, Shamel grunted, and opened his eyes…

"Shamel, I was just thinking. When we go to Maryland to see your brother and Claudine, can we take my car? That long trip will probably be good for it."

Shamel sat up, and thought for a moment.

"Yeah, that will be perfect. I'll leave my car at the precinct, so I won't get any tickets. I can even give you a quick tune-up."

"Great!" Nova replied as they embraced in a hug. "You are the best friend a woman could have!"

"Oh, now I'm just a friend."

"With benefits! Duh!" Nova seductively replied and laughed, but Shamel cut her the *evil-sexy look* with his 'bedroom eyes'. "Uh-oh..." was all Nova said.

People as far north as the Bronx could swear they heard a woman screaming in ecstasy.

Chapter Nineteen

The smell of steak and onions. A baby was crying. The sound of a Sanitation truck backing up to pick up trash. Some couple was having an argument… It was early Saturday morning. Shamel and Nova were preparing for their trip down to Maryland to spend time with Preacher and his family. Shamel carried both overnight bags to the car. Nova came out of the building and stopped in front of Shamel to strike a pose. She was wearing a nice white short set, and looked very stylish. Shamel chose the rugged look, with a T-shirt, blue jeans and sandals. It was a pleasant spring day, with the temperature around 78 degrees. After they got into Nova's Maxima, Shamel remarked, "Flight attendant, prepare for cross-check and take off."

Nova giggled and replied, "Final call for Lover's Airways flight 69 to romance!"

They both laughed, then kissed. Traffic was light. Shamel breezed his way to the George Washington Bridge and onto I-95 headed south. They stopped for gas at the first station along the Jersey Turnpike, then continued on. After passing through the Delaware Memorial Bridge toll, Shamel noticed a stranded male motorist off on the shoulder. Though he wasn't stopping, he did reach for his cell phone on the console to call for assistance, when Nova gently touched his hand, picked up the phone herself and made the call. They smiled at one another. This is how they worked together, oftentimes reading each other's thoughts and sharing the same compassion for helping people. As Shamel neared Laurel, he had Nova dial Preacher just to let him know they were close…

"Haynes residence!" Preacher answered zealously.

"Hi Preach! Just letting you know we're almost there, bro!"

"Hi, Preacher!" Nova chimed in.

"Yo, Nova! What's good, *boo*?"

"Sitting here jamming to WPGC!"

"Yeah, no doubt! We got that on too! Drive safe. I'll see ya when you get here!" Preacher replied.

"Ok, bro, Peace!" Shamel said as Nova disconnected the call.

"Thank you for letting me come." she softly spoke to Shamel.

"Thank you for coming!" he happily replied back.

They gave each other a quick kiss, and held hands for the duration of the trip.

Chapter Twenty

Claudine anxiously waited for Shamel and Nova to arrive. She was in the living room looking out the window while Preacher reclined in his La-Z-Boy reading the newspaper. Suddenly, Claudine became excited…

"They're here! Kids, your uncle's here!" she shouted upstairs to her two children before heading towards the front door. Preacher got up out of the recliner and headed to the door behind Claudine. As Shamel pulled up, he and Nova were having a friendly debate about subway systems…

"I do like the DC Metro stations, but their fare system is strange." Nova said.

"What's really strange is BART – the Bay Area Rapid Transit system. I mean, why in the world would you have an elevated train system in a place where earthquakes occur?" Shamel said. "I *kinda* like CTA myself. You know, Chicago's transit system."

"With all those color-coded charts? Too confusing if you ask me!"

"As long as you can figure out how to get to and from the airports, it's ok. CTA's lines drop you at either 'O'Hare' or 'Midway'. For 'LaGuardia' you still need to catch a bus, and for 'JFK', it will cost you an extra five dollars from the subway."

"Such a shame. We could use that five dollars in Las Vegas."

"So you can lose all your money in the airport slots at 'McCarran' before we even hit the casinos?"

"Whatever! But who needs mass transit when you've got the *Shamel Shuttle*?"

"I'm just happy you know how to drive too!"

Nova looked up towards the house, and saw Claudine standing outside. She immediately waved to her…

"Hi Claudine!"

"Hi, Nova!" – Claudine waved and greeted back. As Nova got out of the car, Claudine approached her with her hands and arms up. Nova met Claudine halfway in the same fashion. They interlocked their hands and squealed with delight before embracing in a hug…

“Oh my god, it’s so good to see you again!” Claudine said to Nova.

“How long has it been? **Too long!**” – they both replied, hugging again.

“Hi Preacher!”

“Nova!” - Preacher exclaimed as they hugged each other.

“Shamel!”

“Preach!” – Shamel said to Preacher as they did the cultural handshake/hug combo.

“Come here, Sha!” – Claudine beamed.

“Hey, Claudine!” Shamel replied as they hugged.

Suddenly without warning, Shamel was accosted by two small forces of energy. Cherelle and Pharaoh, his niece and nephew came bounding out of the house and grabbed a leg each…

“Uncle Sha! Uncle Sha!”- both children shouted vying for Shamel’s attention.

“Hey, get off of me! *Ya always attacking me! Git! Little yard rats!*” – Shamel playfully replied.

“I want a piggy-back ride!” Cherelle said.

"No! Me first!" Pharaoh protested.

"Kids, your uncle and auntie Nova are tired. They will play with you later." Preacher tried convincing both.

"Don't worry. I'll give the both of you rides, but they won't be piggy-back!" Shamel said, as he picked up both children under each arm, to their shrieks of delight.

"Yaa, sack of potatoes!" Cherelle yelled.

"No, football!" Pharaoh yelled out.

"It's football style, Cherelle. *Sack of potatoes* is 'over my shoulder'." Shamel explained.

"Daddy still does that to me!" Cherelle yelled, as both children continued to squeal and giggle with happiness.

"Come on in the house, everyone. Nova, we have so much to do. You know I have to take you to Tysons Corner Center Mall." Claudine said.

"Girl, I don't have a whole lotta money." Nova bashfully replied.

"That's why you need to shop with me! Remember, I have two kids - and a credit limit! Ha!" Claudine replied.

As the two women talked on, Shamel still had the children under his arms. Preacher got the overnight bags from the car, and everyone went inside to prepare for what was destined to be a fun-filled time.

Chapter Twenty-one

A family friend of Preacher and Claudine came by to take the children out from a pre-arranged commitment. This left the adults plenty of time to catch up on each other's lives. Claudine whipped up some tuna sandwiches and iced tea. The four of them was sitting on lawn chairs, engaging in conversation…

"Hey Sha. Tell me about how your names were chosen. I've always been curious." Claudine said.

"Yeah, Sha. You promised me you would elaborate on that." Nova threw in.

"I did, but Preach, do you want to tell them instead?" Shamel asked Preacher.

"Why don't we both tell them?" Preacher replied. He then began…"Our parents met on the same job together in New York City. Dad was from Philly, and mom from Alabama, – **Go figure!" –** Preacher and Shamel both stated. Preacher continued… "Guess it's true what they say about opposites attracting. Here you have a God-fearing, church going woman who wanted no part of 'Blaxploitation'. Yet our father would always rant about being pro-Negro. Don't laugh, I'm serious! What we know as *Afrocentric* today, dad evoked when we were growing up. His all-time favorite scene from a TV show is the scene where the father lifted baby 'Kunta' up to the sky in 'Roots'. Damn. Didn't he do that to us, Shamel?" Preacher reminisced.

"Nope, he did that to you! I wasn't naked!" Shamel chuckled. Nova and Claudine laughed along with him, while Preacher made a face.

"Moving right along," Preacher said, slightly perturbed. "I don't know the reason, but our mother never had a sonogram performed, and didn't realize she was pregnant with twins. She and dad argued over what my name would be-"

"But there were two of you." Nova interrupted.

"Hold on Nova, I'm getting to that." Preacher replied. "Like I said, she had no idea that two of us had been conceived. So when she and Dad reached a compromise, they decided that my name was going to be Preacher Shamel. 'Preacher' for my mother's religious beliefs, and 'Shamel' for my father's 'I'm Black and I'm Proud!' attitude. However, once the doctors realized that my mom had another baby inside her, dad was only too happy to give Shamel the name he wanted me to have after thinking I was his only son and child. So there you have it. I was named Preacher Isaiah…"

"And I was named Shamel Scorpio." Shamel boasted.

"My parents named me Claudine Pamela. What's your middle name, Nova? Claudine asked.

"I don't have one." Nova answered.

"Are you serious?" Claudine pressed.

"Yes. My mom was going to name me Novaline Wilhelmina after my father whose name was William. But, since he decided not to be a part of the equation, she wound up raising me as a single mother. Figuring since he wanted nothing to do with us, she wanted nothing to do with him. Hence, she left only my first name on the birth certificate."

"That's terrible. More men need to step up and handle their responsibility as a father." Claudine fumed.

"I know. Never got a penny of child support from William. She got tired of going to court fighting for it. But we did all right. My grandfather; my mother's father, took up a lot of time with me. I guess I really should say my grandparents. As much as I detest using the word typical, I was the typical child being raised by grandparents because my mother was always working. To her credit though, she went back to school and eventually got a job where she could support the both of us without stress. That, after slaving on two menial jobs to pay for rent, clothes, and food."

"Well, you weren't really raised by your grandparents. They just pitched in to look after you." Shamel said.

"Yeah, Sha, but I grew up without a father. I've never experienced the joy of having 'daddy' take me on his shoulders for a ride, or bike riding. I don't know how it feels to give him a Father's Day card, or have him give me a birthday and Christmas or even a Valentine's Day gift. Thing is, I'll never know. Like Luther Vandross said, 'If I could dance with my father again.' – Humph. We never even so much as bobbed our heads together."

"Right…" - Shamel's voice trailed off. He began to fidget a little, which Preacher noticed right away…

"This tea is good Claudine!" Preacher commented as he took a drink, trying to change the subject. Unfortunately, Claudine didn't pick up on the cue. Totally ignoring Preacher, she said to Nova, "If you could see your father right now, what would you say to him?"

"Nothing. As far as I'm concerned, my mother went through an asexual pregnancy!"

"Don't you mean Immaculate Conception?" Preacher asked.

"No because she had intercourse. Negatively, her relationship to William went on a different course. My mother did date, but she kept her relationships discrete and never exposed me to a lot of men."

At that moment, Shamel got up from the lawn table. While he didn't appear distraught, you can hear it in his voice that all was not well…

"Excuse me; I have to use the bathroom."

"Shamel, are you okay?" Nova asked apprehensively.

"I'm fine! I just have to use the bathroom. Like Preacher said, this is some good tea! Mmm-mmm!"

As Shamel hurried off into the house, Nova turned to Preacher and said, "He barely took a sip. What's wrong with Shamel?"

Preacher gave a deep sigh, then replied, "Shamel never truly got over our father getting killed. He won't admit it, but if he could avenge our father's death he would."

"How are you able to deal with it?" Claudine asked Preacher.

"I don't think about it. No disrespect to my father in anyway, but what's done is done. I used to think if there was some way Shamel and I could mete out revenge on the actual person who took his life, we would. Our mother continued to raise us and our sisters to the best of her ability all alone. Don't get me wrong. I know her caring for me and Shamel on her own made <u>us</u> strong, but there's nothing like having a father figure in your life, especially if you're a boy."

Shamel entered the bathroom, and gently closed the door behind him. He turned on the water, and looked in the mirror. Now his sadness was apparent. Tears streamed out of his eyes as he stood in front of the sink for about a minute. Taking a face cloth, Shamel first wiped his eyes dry, then completely washed his face. He was trying to refrain from his melancholic display, particularly because he didn't want anyone to know how he was truly feeling. Shamel turned off the water and hung the face cloth up when there was a knock on the door…

"Shamel, can I come in?" Nova asked softly.

"I'm coming out now!" Shamel pleasantly replied as if nothing had happened at all. He opened the door, and stood face to face with Nova…

"Are you okay?" she asked.

"Couldn't be better." Shamel answered.

"You sure?"

"Yep. In fact, I'm going outside to get another sandwich."

"I have to use the bathroom myself. I'll be right out." Nova said. Shamel gave Nova a light peck on the lips, then made his way back out to the patio. Neither Preacher nor Claudine brought up the subject of the twins' father again. Instead they made idle chitchat, and when Nova returned, began talking about dieting and weight loss.

Chapter Twenty-two

Shamel grumbled as he looked at the 'Scrabble' board, then looked at his letters and back at the 'Scrabble' board again. Though everyone was playing independently, it was the women versus the men, who possessed a slight lead. But that was about to change. Shamel's face lit up, as he conjured up a word to place in the squares. Leaning over to Preacher, Shamel whispered in his ear, and showed him the letters. Preacher laughed out loud and exclaimed, "You **wiling* (*wilding), but go ahead and use it!" as he gave Shamel a fist bump.

"What are you two plotting? And hurry up Shamel. If you can't make a word, pass!" Claudine snapped.

"Oh – I got your word!" Shamel chortled. He then began singing the theme song from a popular children's show, which Preacher joined in on the chorus…

"I – can – do – anything… Take a look; it's in a book – **'Reading Rainbow'**!"

As he was singing, he slowly and strategically placed the six letters of his word on the 'Scrabble' board. Shamel looked up and flashed a big grin. Nova glared at Shamel as she herself began to sarcastically drone out the theme song to 'Sesame Street'…

"Dat, dat, dat, dat, dat, dat, dat, da-dat! Dat, dat, dat, dat, dat, dat, dat, da-dat..."

Claudine, who at first was staring at the new word Shamel made on the board interrupted her… "Hold it, hold it, hold on, Nova! Shamel, what the hell is that?"

"Jimcrow! As in the 'Jim Crow' laws." Shamel triumphantly said.

"You do know about the 'Jim Crow' laws, don't you honey?" Preacher wisecracked.

"I know about the 'Jim Crow' laws! And that Shamel just cost you fifty points! This isn't 'Ghetto Scrabble'!" Claudine sneered.

Ignoring Shamel and Preacher's pleas for forgiveness, Claudine picked up the pen and tallied up the final score.

"Us, 391! You guys, 324!"

"Serves you right, trying to undermine our intelligence like that!" Nova threw in.

"The kids will be home soon, so I have to get dinner started. But, – ooh! Sometimes you 'X' and 'Y' chromosomes drive me insane!" Claudine huffed.

"Look, we wouldn't be in this mess if that silly *hoe* hadn't eaten from the 'Tree of Knowledge of Good and Evil' in the first place!" Preacher rebuked.

"Who do you think you are, calling someone out of their name?" Claudine replied.

"I'm talking about Eve!"

"I know damn well who you're talking about!"

"Well, Adam should've taken another one of his ribs and beat that witch!" Preacher reasoned.

"Adam was just as culpable! If he had been taking care of business, Eve wouldn't have had to befriend that snake!" Nova disputed.

"Don't blame Adam!" Shamel threw in.

"Yeah, Eve did what you women do all the time!" Preacher asserted.

"Which is?" Claudine challenged.

"Used her charms! Jumped all up in Adam's face with her voluptuous, juicy, robust 'Garden of Eden' body talking *bout*, 'Mmm, take a bite of this, baby!'"

"And just like any other *pussy-whipped* man, Adam's dumb-ass took a bite! If he were a real man, or as you men say, had some *balls,* he would have made Eve throw the rest away, and asked God for some 'Holy Syrup of Ipecac'!"

"You know, you complain about us 'X' and 'Y' chromosomes, but it weren't for **us**, the economy would really suffer!" Preacher said.

"Yeah, cause woman got her game from a man, and they play the game better than us!" Shamel said.

"How do you figure?" Claudine asked.

"Why else are you going to spend your money on weaves and nails? If only women inhabited the planet, looks wouldn't matter!" Preacher inferred.

Both Shamel and Nova let out an "Oooh!", as Claudine prepared to go on the defensive…

"See, Nova? Now they want to join 'Club Chauvinism'! We're going to have to show them why **we** are the better sex!"

"You're taking this too far." Preacher said. "All I meant was-"

"Oh, no, no, no, no, no! If you think you're getting out of this that easily, you wait till you find yourself sleeping in your Jeep! Need proof of who's smarter? I'll give you a good example! Nova, just last week, we were watching 'Biography' on 'A&E'. Barbra Streisand was being profiled. Here Preacher comes way out of left field, asking me this question; 'Didn't Barbra Streisand play in 'Lentil'?' I said to him, 'It's **<u>Yentl</u>**, you idiot!"

Nova and Shamel couldn't contain themselves. They burst out laughing, almost falling to the floor. Preacher felt foolish, and attempted to get even.

"At least **I** didn't mix bleach with ammonia and nearly turn the house into a gas chamber! (Cough, cough!)"

"Everyone makes mistakes. But while I'm calmly opening windows to let the house air out, here you go; '(pant, pant) Dini! Dini! We have to call the fire department! We have to get the kids out! We need oxygen!' - We need oxygen, all right, - 'The Oxygen Network'! Let a female teach you how to be masculine!"

The screams and howls of laughter from Nova and Shamel really irritated Preacher now. He shot back, "You 'Howard' grads are all alike!"

"Psss! You 'Hampton' grads are all alike! And you know full well that my institution of learning has nothing to do with my Intelligence Quotient!" Claudine rebuked.

"I went to 'John Jay College of Criminal Justice' myself." Shamel said.

"Nova, where did you attend college at?" Claudine asked.

"Ow! – 'Syracuse'! That was, up until I received an academic dismissal." Nova replied, somewhat embarrassed.

"Oh no! What happened?" Claudine asked, concerned.

"Girl, I got up there and started partying! Next thing I knew, I wound up going through nearly the entire 'CUNY' system! Bronx, Lehman, City, Baruch, Kingsborough, New York Tech, Medger Evers, and York! I finally ended up at Hunter College, where I managed to escape with an Associate's Degree in Liberal Arts. Guess I should have Sigma, Tau, Upsilon, Delta, Iota, Epsilon, Delta more!" Nova replied, winking at Claudine.

"Huh? What does all that mean?" Shamel asked.

"Don't answer him!" Claudine cut in, winking back at Nova. "You know the Phonetic Alphabet, figure it out!"

"That's Greek, what she just rattled off." Preacher said, a bit perturbed.

"It borders on the same principle! Gee, you guys are getting awfully testy. Feel like conceding now, or shall we continue to punish you?" Claudine replied smugly.

"Why surrender? Nova's the one who barely got through college!" Shamel ridiculed.

"Like Claudine said, it has nothing to do with intelligence!" Nova replied.

"Get him, Nova!" Claudine cheered.

"Oh I'm about to!" Nova answered. "It's true. My GPA suffered a heavy blow. I graduated with a 2.6, but that's only because I was unmotivated and too lazy to do the work. I'll tell you what my dream job is though."

"Let me guess, being the rat at 'Chuck E. Cheese'?" Shamel clowned.

Nova looked at Claudine, and Claudine looked at Nova. Claudine just shook her head, as Nova cracked her knuckles. Staring Shamel in the face, she gave this reply…

"You know how when a plane crashes, it breaks up into various pieces?"

"Yeah…" Shamel replied uneasily. This time, it was Nova who flashed a wide grin and boasted proudly.

"Well, I would be one of those individuals charged with the daunting task of putting it back together again. See, I applied for a job with the NTSB as an Air Safety Investigator - a job that a dumb-ass can't perform. Because I don't possess the appropriate pilot certification, I can't get hired for that. Otherwise, I'd be making more money than you, and we wouldn't be having this conversation!"

"Yeah! That's right girl!" Claudine remarked, clapping her hands and giving Nova a fist bump.

"Man, Sha, your woman is smart! So much for male domination!" Preacher cheerfully sighed.

"Oh, now you want to respect us! Men like you are the reason why women couldn't go to college, vote or receive legal abortions!" Claudine said.

"Hey, I'm all for 'women's lib'!" Shamel insisted.

"Don't even try it! You're a woman hater too!" Nova scolded.

"I'm not gay!"

"I don't mean in that context, you clown!" Nova then turned to Claudine and said, "He's claiming not to be sexist, but this is the same man who believes there's something phallic about 'Ms. Pac-Man' eating all those dots!"

"Oh really? And just what does that make 'Mr. Pac-Man'?" Claudine challenged.

"It doesn't matter. Man gotta eat!" replied Shamel, looking away.

No sooner had he uttered that sentence however, like lightning and without warning, Nova slapped him right upside his head!

"Ow!" Shamel yelled out, as he cut Nova one of the dirtiest looks he could afford, with her returning one in kind. Claudine on the other hand, was ecstatic.

"Thank you Nova, that was well-deserved!" She then turned to Preacher and said, "It's only a matter of time before you get popped upside your *nugget* as well!"

"All right! Don't say nothing when you miss your 'period' next month!" Preacher replied.

The comment stunned Claudine, Nova, and Shamel, who were all momentarily speechless. Shamel started laughing.

"That was rude!" Nova admonished.

Claudine just slowly shook her head and replied, "Not even in fun!" She then said to Nova, "Nova, I love my kids. But after spending seventy-two hours in labor with 'little big head'…"

Shamel composed himself and spoke up; "Okay. I think we played this game long enough!"

"I agree. Come here, baby." Preacher said to Claudine, as he attempted to hug her. But Claudine wasn't having it…

"No! Get away from me! Leave me alone!"

"Claudine!"

"Get away from me, Preacher!"

"Claudine? Oh come on Claudine! I'm sorry!"

"That you are!"

"Claudine?"

"No! See? You're always teasing me!"

"Come on, you know I didn't mean it."

Claudine slowly began to give in to Preacher, as Shamel and Nova both watched and giggled.

"You know I love you." Preacher said.

"No you don't!" Claudine replied.

"Yes, I do!"

"Well then…"

Preacher got a kiss in.

"Well – stop teasing me!"

Nova and Shamel both uttered, "Awww!" as Preacher and Claudine finally embraced and kissed each other.

"You ready to make up with me as well?" Shamel asked Nova.

"Don't know why I should! But then again, you know I love your chauvinistic ass!"

Now Claudine and Preacher went "Awww!" as Nova and Shamel embraced in a kiss.

Just then, the doorbell rang. The kids had finally arrived home after being out with the family friend. Claudine continued to prepare dinner while Preacher went to answer the door. Nova and Shamel got up from the table and decided to go pick up a few items from the store.

Chapter Twenty-three

Cherelle and Pharaoh were playing 'Operation'. Their game playing went very subtle, until Preacher started irking them…

"Hey, can I have a rib bone?"

"No, daddy! It goes to the game!" Cherelle answered.

"But I want that rib. In fact, I want the toes too!"

"Daddy, come on! We're trying to play!"

"Okay. Can I have <u>your</u> toes? I got some toe jam to go with that!"

"MA! Daddy's bothering me and Pharaoh!" Cherelle finally yelled out.

"And he's telling us to eat his icky toe jam!" Pharaoh added.

"Preacher, will you leave my children alone?" Claudine griped.

"Oh sure. They're <u>your</u> children now. But as soon as one of them does something wrong, then they're MY children! Preacher retorted.

"You don't need to be annoying them! Go play with Shamel!"

"Go play with Shamel!" Preacher repeated sarcastically, as he walked off.

"And stop mocking me!" Claudine yelled after him. "Sheesh! I'm telling you Nova, it's like having **three** children sometimes!"

"You don't have to tell me! Shamel acts the same way. We may not have kids, but that is a silly man!" Nova replied.

"Anyway, getting back to what we were talking about. I'm really glad you applied for a government job. By chance, do you have any civil service status?" Claudine asked Nova.

"No. I just kept going back to the 'Jacob Javits' Federal building and worked the kiosk. I guess once I get a stable job somewhere, I'll go back to school and get my bachelor's."

"You could just finish up now. Take 12 credits and you'll be done in no time."

"I don't want to deal with the loans. I was fortunate to get financial aid while I was enrolled, but I'm no longer eligible."

"It's too bad you're not close to the DC area. I can get you in where I work at the Library of Congress."

"Wow! Do you know someone?"

"Nova, I am someone! GS–12, Human Resources!"

"You think Shamel would mind me taking a leave of absence from him?"

"You should! You know you're welcome to stay here."

"It's tempting, but knowing Sha, he would miss me too much. I know I sure would miss him!"

"Look, you want to be financially independent and secure. Now you could take your chances with 'Powerball', if you don't mind spending a dollar or two every week. My point is, tangible is best. Nova, you're very smart, educated, and young. Hopefully you and Sha will build a life together. I'm not just saying that because he's my brother-in-law. I honestly think you two make a really nice couple. But, don't ever trade in your independence for co-dependency."

"I hear everything you're saying, but I'm co-dependent right now – at least till I find a decent paying full-time job!"

Claudine shifted her position in her chair, and unfolded her arms, bringing them in front of her. At that moment, Nova caught a good glimpse of Claudine's wedding ring. It was huge. It was very huge. It was a 3 carat platinum marquise diamond solitaire bridal set. For an instant, Nova became very envious. She didn't know how she hadn't noticed it before, but was certainly paying attention to it now! Claudine caught Nova glancing at her ring, and decided to pay heed…

"Do you like this?"

"Well, yes! Nova exclaimed.

"Here's a good example of the type of independence I'm trying to stress to you, Nova. When Preacher and I went shopping for our rings, I said to him, 'Choose what you like and I'll purchase it.' And this set was *banging*, I've got to admit! I make good money, so price was never an issue. We work in symmetry, where I'll cover some things, and he'll cover others. But we also work as an entity, and come together as one for all. This isn't a reflection on Preacher in anyway, but if he wasn't in my life, I would do all right by myself. Gotta admit, though we have our little differences, I love that man, and wouldn't trade him for all the diamond and platinum rings still being mined in Africa! You have a good man too, and I know Shamel will do right by you."

"Yeah. He fusses at me, and I get on him, but we always manage to come together at the same point. It's great when you can see eye to eye most of the time on things that matter, instead of one person believing their word is law, and you have no say in your defense."

"I agree."

At that moment, Pharaoh entered the kitchen. He tapped Claudine on her leg and said, "Mommy, can I get some ice cream please?"

"May I have some ice cream, please?" Claudine corrected him.

"May I have some ice cream, mommy?" Pharaoh correctly asked.

"Yes, you may." Claudine answered.

"Thank you." Pharaoh replied.

As Pharaoh went to the freezer to get the ice cream, the women continued their conversation. He opened the door to reach for the ice cream, then closed it again and walked back over to Claudine's chair.

"Mommy?"

"Yes, sweetie?"

"There's no more ice cream." Pharaoh whimpered.

A look of surprise came over Claudine's face. She turned to Nova and exclaimed, "That was almost a new half-gallon!" Claudine then turned towards the living room area and yelled, "Preacher? PREACHER!"

Preacher however couldn't hear her. He was too busy trying to beat Shamel in 'NBA Jam' on the Sony PlayStation 2 set.

"Ah, here it comes! Pippin to Jordan for the 'three'!" Preacher bellowed, as he furiously worked the controller. Shamel was equally as boisterous…

"Ooh! Shot blocked by Sprewell! Rebound-"

"And the steal! Jordan fakes – and BOOM! Ho! Slam dunk! Chicago wins, 107-104!"

Preacher stood up and began doing the 'Harlem Shake' dance. He was being very smug, and about to rub his victory in Shamel's face… "In the words of Marv Albert…"

"Preacher, you greedy pig!" Claudine said loudly, very vexed.

Preacher was caught off guard. With a surprised look on his face, he said to Claudine, "That's not what Marv would say!"

"No, I'm saying it! Preacher, how could you?" Claudine asked, as she viewed the evidence. Two nearly empty bowls of Vanilla Fudge ice cream sat on the coffee table. She became even more riled as Shamel put another spoonful into his mouth, right in front of her. "Between you and 'baby Huey' here, I couldn't even offer Nova any ice cream!"

"There wasn't that much left." Preacher pleaded.

"And who you calling 'baby Huey'?" Shamel retorted.

"You!" Claudine answered.

"Actually, they both look like the 'Michelin tire man'!" Nova threw in.

"Preacher, I want you to go and get these children some more ice cream. Besides, I still need a few items from the supermarket anyway that I wrote on a list. So come on before it gets too late, 'Hardcastle and McCormick'."

"More like 'Tenspeed and Brownshoe'!" Nova giggled. She then whispered into Claudine's ear, and both of them said out loud, "**Crockett and Tubbs!**"

Shamel began to pout at the name-calling but Preacher just took it in stride. He patted Shamel on the shoulder and said, "Let's go, 'Tubbs'!"

"I'm 'Crockett', you're 'Tubbs'!" Shamel shot back.

Preacher went to the hall closet and took out a hooded jacket. "Hold on a moment." he said to Shamel, as he disappeared into the bedroom. Claudine and Nova went back into the kitchen to resume talking. Claudine yelled out to Shamel, "Look on the dining room table. I left the list there!"

Shamel went and picked the list up, glanced at it quickly, then placed it in his pocket. Once Preacher emerged from the bedroom, he said to Shamel, "I'm ready." and they both headed out of the house. Preacher took a key remote out of his pocket, and disarmed the alarm on a Crystal Red Tint coat Cadillac XTS sitting in the driveway. Shamel stopped short and asked Preacher, "Where's the Jeep?"

"In the garage. Claudine and I switched vehicles while I'm on vacation. Said she could use the extra space to run her errands."

Shamel nodded his head in agreement. They both got in the Cadillac. Preacher pumped up the volume on the radio, and off they drove, headed towards DC.

Chapter Twenty-four

Most of the stores where Preacher lived closed early. It was easier to head into DC where he knew things were open, rather than drive around looking. Preacher and Shamel first went to the supermarket to obtain the last few items Claudine needed. Incredibly, they forgot the ice cream. While heading back to the house, Preacher decided to stop at "Bar at Home", a small independent liquor store he patronized whenever he was in *the hood*. As he drove up in front of the store, Preacher was oblivious to the police cruiser that had pulled across the street from them, with the two officers inside watching very intently.

"I'll be right back." Preacher said to Shamel, who nodded his head in acknowledgment.

Preacher entered the store to a melody of jingling from the metal door chime. He made eye contact with and gave *the nod* to a black male that was inside the store playing Lotto, who returned the greeting. Preacher didn't immediately see the owner, so he called out,

"Darren, you around?"

"Be right there!" a voice yelled back. Before long, an elderly yet spry gentleman ambled from a back room. He used a cane to assist him with his gait but was otherwise moving well under his own power.

"Hey Youngblood! Whatcha say?" the elderly man said to Preacher.

"Hi Darren! You know I'm here for the usual." Preacher replied, as he walked around in the aisles, picking up a bottle of Sour Apple Schnapps, Bailey's, Jim Beam 'Devil's Cut', and Strawberry Daiquiri mix. "My brother's in town, so I'll get a bottle of Amaretto as well."

"People like you are the reason why prohibition was repealed. Helps keep my old butt in business!" Darren chortled.

"Well, you just make sure you keep that number for 'A.A.' handy!" Preacher quipped.

He took a $100 bill out of his wallet while Darren rang up the order.

"You know, your bills are the only bills I don't check." Darren said.

"Aw, I feel so special!" Preacher replied.

Then before Darren gave Preacher his change, he took the $100 bill and held it up to the light.

"Yep, it's real!" he said, laughing.

Preacher just shook his head and said, "Man, you too much! By the way, I like that Jersey!" referring to the football Jersey Darren was wearing.

"My grandson got it for me!" Darren said proudly.

"Glad he got the team right!"

At that point, Darren's facial expression turned serious. He leaned over the counter and said to Preacher, "When you gonna stop playing games and become a 'Redskins' fan?"

"Oh no! I've told you before; I'm 'Baltimore Ravens' all day! 'New York Giants' as an alternate!"

"Backstabber! You don't live in New York anymore!"

"Doesn't matter. My brother still does, and when his team is winning, I have to give him my full support!"

"You 'dunkis'! Maybe if they got rid of that *gopher boy* – what's his name," Darren pondered, snapping his fingers. "What the hell is his name? Oh well! Anyway if they get rid of him, they could actually win some games!"

"You mean Terrence Mole?"

"Yeah! That's it!"

"Hell, Terrence is the best Running Back to be drafted yet!" Preacher argued.

"You gonna stand there and tell me he's better than Bo Jackson, Herschel Walker, Emmitt Smith, or Tony Dorsett? Mourn!" Darren replied, making his cheeks quiver.

"Hey, it's just like the 'Virginia Warlocks'. They've been *hurting* for a good Quarterback ever since Sam 'speedball' Comesidan retired, and he's the best there was!"

"You kidding me? Even <u>he</u> wasn't that good! Always on the injured reserve list! I know Junior varsity players that are tougher <u>and</u> better than him! See Youngblood, your problem is you don't know your history. Try watching old footage from the USFL archives, then come and talk to me!

A lot of these new boys are over-rated, yet they get these million-dollar endorsements tossed at them like rice being thrown at a wedding. Then they let you down by failing to at least make the playoffs!"

"Getting back to Terrence Mole, he has an impressive record. I'd say his stats rival that of many of these Hall of Famers!" Preacher defended.

"How many *Heisman*'s did he earn?"

"Uh, not sure?"

"Try zero! How many *Lombardi*'s did he win?"

Preacher was speechless. Darren stood erect, slapped the counter with his hand and declared,

"I rest my case!"

Once again, Preacher felt foolish. He looked for a means of gaining leverage. After glancing around and spying a particular brand of liquor on the counter, he said, "You ever been hit with a bottle of 'Cherry Kijafa'?"

Darren's eyes widened in surprise, and he replied, "No, but I'll tell you what. I'm gonna make you disappear. Cause just like that rap song says, 'I got the magic stick'! Now get the hell out of my store!"

Upon that, he picked up his cane and swung it at Preacher, purposely missing him. It was enough to send Preacher scrambling though, as he grabbed the bag of liquor and high-tailed it to the door. Laughing, Preacher said, "Okay Darren, take care!"

"You too, Youngblood! See you again soon!"

Preacher exited and hopped back into the Cadillac, placing the bag of liquor on the back seat. He put the car in gear, and began driving off. That's when the police cruiser that had been across the street from him and Shamel made a U-turn, and began following them.

"Darren's crazy! He threatened me, you know!" Preacher jovially bemoaned to Shamel.

"Oh? Do tell!" Shamel replied.

"We always get into it about sports. Somehow he always manages to get one up on me, no matter which sport we debate!"

Shamel laughed, but just as Preacher was going to continue telling him about the face-off with Darren, he took notice to the police cruiser tailing them.

"Hey Sha, I think we're being followed."

Shamel looked in the passenger mirror, and then commented, "Another 'driving while black' scenario?"

"I'm not sure. Let me make this *right*."

Preacher signaled, slowed, and made a right turn. Sure enough, the police cruiser made the turn as well.

"Hmmm. Okay. Let's have some fun. By chance, do you have your *piece* with you?" Preacher said to Shamel.

"No, I left it in the house." Shamel replied.

"Open the glove compartment."

Shamel opened the glove compartment and exclaimed, "Ooh!" as he took out a Beretta 21 Bobcat .22-caliber pistol.

"I went in the room to grab my service firearm. Not that I expected trouble or anything, but that gun there I just picked up for my new backup weapon. Took it to the range which is why it was in the car to begin with." Preacher explained to Shamel.

"I think it's time to give these cops what they deserve!" Shamel said to Preacher, as he put the pistol in his waistband.

"I agree. Racial profiling is going to end tonight – with us! Just follow my lead."

"Got it."

"Oop! They just lit us up! Here we go!"

Preacher signaled, and pulled over as the police cruiser, now with its dazzle lights, flashers, and blinding spotlights within the light bar signaled for them to stop. Both Preacher and Shamel sat motionless, but they were smirking the entire time. Finally after about thirty seconds, both officers, one white and the other black, got out and approached the car. The driver approached Preacher's side, with his firearm out. The other officer approached Shamel's side with his weapon still holstered, but his hand at the ready. Preacher took notice that they were with the Sheriff's department, and one of the agencies' community programs. He had already lowered the window, and was waiting for the Sheriff to speak…

"Nice car. Did you borrow it from the neighborhood?" the sheriff said to Preacher in a condescending tone. "License, registration and insurance."

"Good evening, Sgt. Don't I even get a 'Hello Sir' or some other form of acknowledgment?" Preacher asked.

The sheriff gave Preacher a very stern look, then said, "I won't ask you again - sir."

"Well, I do have a right to know why I was pulled over. Besides, you seem like you're ready to play 'Tin Pan Alley', so before I go reaching for any credentials, I think it's fair to ask you 'if I may?', as my wallet is in my pocket. **I certainly wouldn't want you to think I had a gun**."

Preacher purposely spoke aloud now, turning his head and winking at Shamel, who supplemented with,

"Yeah. **Cause you gotta have a carry permit, in order to carry.**"

Both cops seemed unimpressed. The one on Preacher's side then said, "Out of the car with your hands where I can see them, and we'll let you boys know why you were stopped."

"I feel rather uncomfortable with your gun already out. Couldn't you at least tell me now why we were pulled over?" Preacher said to the sheriff.

"We have a stolen vehicle report with a car matching this exact description. So before I charge you with resisting arrest, you better get your ass out of this car!" the sheriff responded.

Preacher slapped the dashboard, and said, "Will ya look at that? We went from show your credentials, to being arrested on suspicion of grand theft-auto! Okay, you got me! Might as well arrest my accomplice too. He's the one who decided not to go for the convenience store!"

"Don't blame me! You said your feet were hurting!" Shamel threw in.

As Preacher exited the Cadillac, Shamel began to get out as well.

"Freeze! Stay in the car!" the deputy on his side of the car barked, unholstering his weapon.

"Be easy, *brother*! You have to understand. We're like Siamese twins. He don't go nowhere without me, and I don't go nowhere without him!" Shamel stated, as he continued getting out.

"I said stay put! I'm not your brother – ***brother!*** Save that hip-hop plea bargaining for the music video!" the deputy on Shamel's side yelled.

Preacher stepped in again…

"Look, he's gotta stretch his legs. If he doesn't, they'll cramp up, and you'll have a medical emergency on your hands."

"Yeah. I got that spine-of-beef eater thing going on. It travels down to my sciatic nerve, makes me twitch."

Upon that, Shamel pushed his way out of the Cadillac. The deputy now had his weapon fully drawn and trained on Shamel.

"You people don't know how to listen! Turn around and place your hands on the car!" he yelled at Shamel. Shamel turned around and complied.

"You put your hands on the damn car also, homey!" the sheriff who had Preacher confronted said to him.

"Gee, now I'm a 'homey'. This just gets better and better." Preacher said, as he turned around and put both his hands on the roof of the car.

"Yeah, looks like you homeboys picked the wrong hood to be chilling in!" the deputy sheriff dealing with Shamel said.

The sheriff with Preacher began a pat down.

"Got any weapons on you?"

"I do have one weapon of mass destruction - my weapon of **ass** destruction!"

He and Shamel laughed, just as the sheriff found Preacher's service pistol.

"GUN!" he yelled to his partner, as he pulled it out and tossed it to the ground.

"Hey, I got one of those!" Shamel quipped, upon which he was immediately patted down. As soon as the deputy sheriff found Shamel's pistol in his waistband he too yelled out "GUN!" and immediately tossed it to the ground.

"You're both under arrest!" the sheriff dealing with Preacher said, as he pulled out a pair of handcuffs. "Place your hands behind your head!" he ordered Preacher.

At that moment, Preacher did something very risky that could have cost him his life. He immediately put both of his hands in his pockets, then turned around and faced the sheriff. The sheriff stepped back, and aimed his gun right at Preacher's chest.

"Hands out of your pockets now or I'll shoot! I'll kill you, you-"

"Black *whatever you're gonna say*?" Preacher interrupted, cutting the sheriff off. "Before you say another word, check my credentials!"

Upon that, Preacher cautiously withdrew his wallet with his right hand. He tossed it at the sheriff, who caught it with one hand. Shamel turned to the deputy sheriff holding the gun on him and said, "You need to check mine as well." He slowly put his hand in his right pocket, and slowly removed his wallet, which he handed to the deputy sheriff.

"Stay put or else! I'm watching you!" he snarled at Shamel.

Keeping his gun trained on Shamel, he moved around to the driver's side of the Cadillac with the Sgt. Both of them opened each wallet - and looked in disbelief at the ID and mini police shield displayed in the holders. The deputy sheriff who had subdued Shamel swallowed hard. He then hesitantly remarked to the Sgt., "New York? These are fake."

"The sheriff who had subdued Preacher glanced at Shamel's wallet, and commented, "No, they're not. This is a Virginia police shield. Put your gun down." as he holstered his own weapon.

Shamel walked around and joined Preacher on the driver side of the Cadillac. Both sheriffs shamefully handed the wallets back to Preacher and Shamel. The sheriff who accosted Preacher then spoke.

"Detective, I'm - we're truly sorry. We had no idea that you were who you are, and we hope you understand."

"Um-hum." Preacher replied, nodding his head with his arms folded. "You know, normally, I'd let this slide. However, Sgt. 'Norcon', it seems to me that you are teaching this **rookie**, who coincidentally is named deputy 'Eagle', not how to soar like one, but instead be unprofessional, judgmental, and downright rude!"

"Don't forget insensitive and bigoted!" Shamel added.

"You didn't even bother to state that this is a known drug area. I know you didn't run the plate by the way you addressed me in this **nice car.** Had it been stolen, you would have had half the precinct come out for us! Auto theft is not even part of your job assignment, which says to me that you were looking for two *niggers to serve*, instead of protect."

"Some cops ought to be downright ashamed of themselves!" Shamel said, glaring at Deputy Eagle.

"I would remove that American Flag pin from your lapel and replace it with a Confederate one. You were also unaware that I am an Instructor Trainer for officers in the *D.A.R.E. (*Drug Abuse Resistance

Education) program in this region. But you won't have that privilege to abuse your authority anymore. I want your shields."

"Oh come on! There's no need to-" Sgt. Norcon began to protest, until he was abruptly cut off by Preacher heatedly demanding,

"I want your shields, NOW!"

"Yes, sir!" they meekly replied, quickly handing over their badges to Preacher.

"Deputy Eagle, would you kindly hand me your pen and pad? I'm taking notes this time." Preacher said to the deputy, who listlessly turned over his notepad and a pen to Preacher who then began to jot down their information…

"Who's your commanding officer?" Preacher asked both sheriffs. Deputy Eagle shuffled his feet, then said, "Sgt. Norcon is my superior while I'm still training."

"Like I asked, who is your C.O.?" Preacher said again, more sternly.

The Sgt. sighed, then answered "Sheriff Beasley."

"Alfonso Beasley? Oh man. You guys are really in trouble. Would you two mind doing me a favor? Please tell **Al**, I apologize for not getting back to him in a timely fashion, but my family and I would love to attend his annual 4th of July barbecue **again** this year. Hey Shamel, you and Nova can come too if you like!"

"Consider my 'holiday request off' already submitted!" Shamel enthusiastically replied.

Preacher wrote down both of the sheriff's names, badge numbers, and their county office. After tearing off the sheet he wrote on, he handed the deputy back the notepad and pen, then said to both of them, "When you get back, make sure you tell your watch commander that **Detective Haynes** is the one who put you out of service. I'm sure whoever it is knows me quite well. Don't worry about giving him a reason, because I'll be by in the morning to file a formal complaint. Have a good night."

Shamel put his left hand under his chin and wiggled his fingers at them, sarcastically remarking "Buh-bye!" to both sheriffs. Without saying another word or looking back at Preacher and Shamel, they get into their cruiser, turned off the dazzle, flashers, and spotlight, and drove away. The brothers watched as they drove away, and when the tail lights disappeared from view, rejoiced in the moment.

"You do realize that was some dumb 'ish' we just pulled!" Shamel exclaimed as he picked up and handed Preacher his gun, then walked around the Cadillac to retrieve the other.

"I know! I need a drink behind that!" Preacher snorted.

Preacher opened the back door of the Cadillac and took out the Bourbon and Amaretto. He opened the *Devil's Cut* for himself, then opened the Amaretto for Shamel.

"Uh, Preach?" Shamel said, a bit apprehensive.

"Look Sha, I could have been killed. And you know they would've did you too, because dead men don't talk!"

"True indeed!" Shamel admitted. He then took the Amaretto from Preacher and held it up, as Preacher prepared to make a toast.

"To us. For being law-abiding citizens – as well as some *brothers* with some rank!"

"Cheers!" Shamel said, as they gently clinked the bottles together.

Both of them took healthy swigs from the bottles, with Preacher making a face and exclaiming "Whew!" and Shamel uttering "Ahh!" before recapping them. Shamel then took the Bourbon from Preacher, and placed both bottles in the back seat with the others again.

"Let's go home, bro! You know the women ain't going to believe this one!" Preacher asserted. Just before he drove off, he turned to Shamel and asked, "By the way, you did mean *spina bifida*, right?"

Preacher and Shamel cracked up with hilarity, as Preacher sped off towards home. As soon as they got in though, without giving them the opportunity to explain or defend themselves, Claudine chewed them out for taking such a long time.

"And you mean to tell me, that after all this time you still forgot the ice cream?" Claudine seethed.

Preacher and Shamel looked at each other, and then Shamel innocently replied,

"It wasn't on the list."

Chapter Twenty-five

Stefan pulled up into the parking area of American University, where Mstislab was already situated awaiting his arrival. Mstislab was standing outside his vehicle with the windows down, and as usual was enjoying a cigarette. Stefan approached Mstislab with a female companion in tow, but also noticed that Seryoga was in the vehicle with him…

"Who's your *Blad (*Whore)?" Mstislab questioned abrasively.

"Just a friend. We were on our way to a motel when you called."

"What dedication! He decided to do me before getting done!"

"Just wait for me in the car, I won't be too long." Stefan said to his female companion who complied, yet stayed silent the entire time.

"So Mstislab, any particular reason why we're here on the campus of American University at 0200 hours which is about as risky as swimming in shark infested waters?"

"Symbolism. But let's talk inside my mobile office."

Seryoga was sitting in the passenger seat. He got out to allow Stefan to sit, and went to get in the back seat when Mstislab stopped him.

"Seryoga, I need a few moments with Stefan alone."

"I thought I always sat in on conferences." Seryoga disputed.

"Well, you're not sitting in on this one."

"Any reason why?"

"Because I said so." Mstislab answered in a monotone, void of emotion. Stefan looked at Seryoga, and Seryoga glared at Stefan. Seryoga then slowly exited the vehicle firmly closing the door behind him. As he walked away, Mstislab and Stefan began talking.

"He didn't look too pleased, Mstislab."

"He'll be fine. It's like I told you and everyone else back at the Marriott. I'm making lots of changes. I'm sure you want the 'American dream' as much as I do. If my plan is going to come to fruition, these changes are very necessary. Jaska and Nunchaku have already been reassigned. Seryoga doesn't know it yet, but I'm sending him to do a *hit* in Maryland on another brigadier that's been screwing up. This is where you come in. I'm giving more responsibility to you now, in addition to your second chance. I know you have that information I requested."

"I won't let you down this time. But I thought that Thomas was going to be here too, just to verify things."

"Thomas had duty and couldn't make it, but he assured me that all of what he gave you is accurate. Though I did not do formal introductions, we're bringing on board a lot of naval personnel, which includes some of my former shipmates from the Russian Navy. All of these people were at the meeting in Philadelphia."

"Well, here's the rundown. Most of the ships are going to the 34th St. West side pier by the Intrepid. That's where all of the security and heavy police presence will be. Our stuff is with the '*Pegasus* Carrier Group'. The actual transport is the USS Minotaur. Thomas assured me, that ship is going to the Brooklyn Marine terminal for docking."

"They better, because even South Street Seaport has too much police activity!"

"You don't want the Seaport. Too close to downtown Manhattan and not secluded enough."

"That's why what I'm about to impose on you is so important."

Mstislab leaned into Stefan, and looked him straight in his eyes.

"I want **you**, to *head up* Boston. I gave it much thought, and decided that you are the best one for this task."

Stefan sat silent for a moment. He then flashed a broad grin and replied, "I guess I can learn to like the Celtics! By the way, you like to gamble, right?"

"Of course!"

"I heard there are some casinos outside of Boston. After things get situated up there, we need to go hit a few!"

"I knew I picked the right man for this job!" Mstislab exclaimed, as he engaged Stefan in a one armed hug.

"What happens now?" Stefan asked.

"We go to New York for Fleet Week. Because we need to be there, I've purposely been slowing things down here in DC, and I plan to shut this down for a while."

"You're not serious!"

"I don't mean I'm closing up shop forever. Too much money being made for that! However, I can't be in two places at once, nor do I have the manpower with everyone scrambling to get the Boston operation off the ground. Once we have Boston on lockdown, I'll head back this way, and get in touch with my Florida contacts. We're on our way to becoming the strongest and largest cartel on the Eastern seaboard. No one - and I do mean no one, will be able to stop us! For me, it's about capitalism. While I will keep our Russian mafia all Russian, I will continue to forge alliances, allegiances, and connections with people who will help us mirror the same structure, power, and muscle that was depicted in 'The Godfather'..."

Mstislab paused for a moment to light up another cigarette, then continued as Stefan just listened attentively…

"You know, not a whole lot of people can say they actually read the novel. Sure everyone saw the movies. But until you read; until you get in the writer's head; you cannot begin to appreciate, understand, and see what it is that is truly being said. *Puzo* is a genius! Thanks to technology and fear, *M.A.D.* is going to be a mafia family which will be feared and revered - for years!"

"Mad? I don't understand." Stefan stated.

"My namesake. My initials, Stefan. **M** - **M**sti**slav**, **A** - **A**fanasi, **D** - **D**iviodich. I don't want to be known just as Russian mafia. I have everyone refer to me as **Msti-slab.** 'Slab' for short, because a slab is where anyone who defies me ends up. We need an image and a name. So that's it. The more notorious we become, the more power we will acquire! You good with this?"

"Yes, we're good. Just curious. What are you going to do about Seryoga?"

"Ser-who?"

Mstislab and Stefan laughed out loud. But unbeknownst to Mstislab, Seryoga had walked back near the Hummer within earshot of their voices and heard that last comment about him. Though Seryoga didn't say a word nor let on that he'd overheard what was said, it would definitely stick with him in his mind.

"Seryoga is still the point man for getting everyone with those weapons to Boston. All goes well; we should meet up at the same time so I don't have to…"

Mstislab looked up, and noticed Seryoga close by.

"Seryoga! Come on back. We're done."

"All right Mstislab, I'll be talking to you." Stefan said, as he gave Mstislab a fist bump before getting out of the Hummer. He smiled and nodded his head at Seryoga, who darted his eyes keep from looking at him.

"Stefan, one more thing!" Mstislab yelled after him. Stefan paused and turned around with an inquisitive look on his face.

"Think your lady friend might be interested in a threesome?" Mstislab asked eagerly.

"She might be interested, but I'm not." Stefan replied.

"Fine then. I'll talk to you later."

As Stefan made his way back to his car, Seryoga finally got back into the front passenger seat of the Hummer, but kept his head down. He had no intention of showing his displeasure to Mstislab.

"What's the matter with you?" Mstislab asked Seryoga.

"Nothing. Just tired."

"You better rest up, because I have an errand for you to run, and I mean **you**. No more delegating to someone else. Since I'm tired myself, I'll give you the details later. We're crashing at the safehouse till morning. You'll head out from there."

"Works for me, 'Slab'."

Seryoga said it with such indifference, that Mstislab cut him a look, but Seryoga kept his head down and didn't pay any mind. When Seryoga did finally look up, he kept his gaze directed out the window, as Mstislab drove off towards the safehouse to rest for the night, Euro Dance music blasting away.

Chapter Twenty-six

Nova awoke before anyone else in the house. She got up to use the bathroom, then decided to check her email. Since arriving at Preacher and Claudine's home, she hadn't been on the internet, and had quite a bit of mail to go through. She had gone through about twenty emails for job responses when she clicked on the next one. First, Nova quickly scanned it, and then she read it again slowly from the beginning. Excitedly, she jumped up and scurried back into the bedroom where Shamel was still sleeping.

"Shamel! Shamel!" Nova loudly whispered as she gently shook Shamel.

"Huh? There a break-in?" he asked with sleep in his voice.

"No! Guess what? I got a job interview!"

Shamel yawned and sat up. Rubbing the sleep out of his eyes, he replied "That's great! Congratulations baby! When's the interview?"

"It's tomorrow. Oh, wow! That means we have to go back to New York! I'm sorry Sha, I didn't mean to cut your trip short!"

"First off, you have nothing to apologize for. Second and please don't take this personal, but I don't have to go back with you. It's <u>your</u> car."

"True, but how are you going to get back?"

"You know me. Greyhound, Megabus, Amtrak, rickshaw. I'll figure it out!"

"Are you sure?"

"Listen Nova. You've been waiting a long time for a decent job to come through. It may not be exactly what you want, but like I always say, a little bit of something – beats a whole lot of nothing!"

Nova hugged Shamel, then kissed him on the lips.

"I better go freshen up, then start packing."

"I'll go wake 'the Haynes' and let them know you have to leave."

"I thought we were the 'Haynes'."

"No. See, we're the 'Haynes-Springfield's'. You haven't been converted."

"Could I keep my last name, if such a conversion were to take place?"

"Maybe. Luckily for you, they actually sound nice together!"

"Well, 'Springfield-Haynes' sounds better, but I'll take what I can get!"

Nova then began to get her things together, while Shamel went to inform Preacher and Claudine of her departure.

Chapter Twenty-seven

Later that morning, Nova was all packed and ready to go. She was giving her final goodbyes to Cherelle and Pharaoh, Preacher and Claudine.

"Girl, good luck on that interview! I know you'll get this job!" Claudine hummed.

"I hope. I'm optimistic, but I'm still going to be a bit of a pessimist till they say I'm hired!"

Nova got into her car. Shamel stood by the driver's side door and bent down to give her one last kiss, as well as something else…

"Hey Nova. I was actually going to give this to you once we got back in New York, but since you're leaving me prematurely…"

"Oh, stop it! What do you have for me?" Nova cooed.

Shamel reached into his pocket and pulled out a small black velvet covered box. He opened it to reveal an 18k gold charm in the shape of a NYC Detective's shield with a chain. Embedded within the charm was Shamel's badge number.

"Oh Sha! When did you get this?" Nova gasped.

Shamel took it out of the box, and placed it around Nova's neck as she leaned forward.

"Remember that day we all went to Tysons Corner and I snuck off with Preacher? This one gold shop actually made it on the spot for me! I figured I'd give it to you now, so, you know – in case you happen to be going a little fast and get stopped."

"Don't worry. I learned <u>how</u> to speed from the best! I love this! I really do, and I love you. Thank you."

"You're welcome." Shamel replied, as they engaged in one final kiss… "Call me as soon as you get in, and be careful."

"I will. Bye."

"Bye."

Shamel, Preacher, and Claudine all waved to Nova as she drove away. Once she was out of sight, Preacher said to Shamel, "Ready to head over to the precinct? I want to get this report filed."

"Sure."

"Now I trust that the two of you will stay out of trouble right?" Claudine mused.

"Well D*ini*, I don't think we can get into much trouble today. But just to be safe, I'm taking **my** vehicle!"

"And I'm getting my firearm!" Shamel said.

"You know, both of you need to become chefs or something!" Claudine replied.

"Oh sure. Stop - in the name of the 'Ginsu'!" Shamel scoffed.

"Boy, don't you mock me! You ain't too big to be slapped, and I will cut you!" Claudine scolded.

"Yeah, and I'm not helping you!" Preacher chided.

"Cause you know I'll slap you too!" Claudine said to Preacher.

"Woman, just go get my car key!"

"I love you Preacher!"

"Yeah? I can't tell!"

Preacher and Claudine continued fussing at one another as usual, while he and Shamel headed back in the house to grab their things. Soon, Preacher and

Shamel were on their way. After arriving at the precinct, they went inside to Preacher's desk to fill out the paperwork.

"How come you don't have your own office?" Shamel ribbed Preacher.

"Do you have your own?" Preacher replied.

"I'm not inside long enough to make use of one."

"So *whatchu* saying? I don't spend enough time pounding the pavement?"

"Well 'Ollie', you do look a bit portly." Shamel snickered.

"Ok 'Stanley', don't get your ass kicked while you're here!" Preacher retorted.

As Preacher and Shamel continued upheaval with one another, two well-dressed Caucasian males came into the precinct. One had no tie on with the top two buttons of his shirt open under his suit jacket, and the other one had shirt and tie intact. They stopped at the information desk, and were directed over to where Preacher and Shamel were sitting. Preacher and Shamel both looked up inquisitively.

"Are you Detective Haynes?" the male with no tie asked, directing the question toward Shamel.

Shamel looked at Preacher who intervened.

"We both are. Which Detective Haynes are you looking for?"

The first male looked at Shamel again, and queried, "Preacher?"

Preacher himself again spoke up, and stated, "He's the altar boy, and I'm the priest!"

"Ha-ha. You better hope they're not from the corny joke squad!" Shamel scolded.

Both of the males took out their wallets simultaneously, and displayed their federal shields. The first male then introduced the two of them.

"Hi. I'm Special agent King; this is Special agent Elvis, NCIS."

"Believe me; we've heard all the jokes." Special agent Elvis stated.

Preacher then said, "Well guys, if this is about that email scam seeking donations for military dependent spouses who's combat wounded husbands need for their home to be modified, I must inform you that 'PayPal' is looking into it, and I have not received any further correspondence from them."

Special agents King and Elvis first gave each other a dumbfounded look, then turned to Preacher with an even more perplexed gaze. Shamel burst out laughing, while Preacher tried to regain his poise.

"Ok, now that I've choked down my piece of humble pie, how can I help you gentlemen?"

"Detective, we were hoping you could help shed some light on a criminal investigation that we're actively pursuing involving naval personnel." Special agent King said.

"I'm somewhat flattered that you would seek my help, but I just so happen to be on vacation. Also, what assistance could I possibly provide you?" Preacher asked.

"Your name was referred to us by a Lieut. Merriweather, from the DC Metro police. He mentioned that you participated in a raid with him on a purported safehouse. This safehouse was referred to in a written confession by a seaman we now have in custody. We have no intention of taking up all of your time, but if you would be kind enough to come back to NCIS headquarters for an interview, it would be greatly appreciated. We'll also see to it that you're dropped back here at your precinct."

"Okay, I have no problem with that. By the way, this is my twin brother, Detective Shamel Haynes, NYPD."

Shamel extended his hand to shake Special Agent King's... "Pleasure to meet you, agent King."

"Please, call me Tristian. My partner, Zachary Elvis."

"Pleasure to meet you as well." Agent Elvis said to Shamel, extending and shaking his hand.

"I'm ready if you're ready." Preacher said to Tristian.

"Great. Let's go." Tristian replied.

All four men filed out of the precinct into a dark blue sedan with US government license plates. Agent King got into the driver's seat, and drove off towards NCIS headquarters back in Washington.

Chapter Twenty-eight

The Washington Navy Yard was bustling with activity. Security was tight at the front gate, with both heavily armed civilian guards and military police performing strict ID and vehicle checks. Agent King was waved through after displaying his ID to one of the guards. He pulled into a spot marked "Reserved for NCIS Agents only", and the four of them exited the vehicle. The offices of NCIS were brightly lit and full of the sounds of a busy workplace. Phones were ringing, computers humming, photocopiers and document shredders were performing their functions. Agent King directed Preacher and Shamel towards a door that had his name and title outside on the wall: Tristian King, NCIS Special Agent. Upon entering the room, both Preacher and Shamel were impressed at the décor. It was a spacious office, with two chairs in front of a big desk. There were plants around the room. On the desk were various photos in frames. Preacher figured that the pictures of a woman with three children were Tristian's family. What really caught his attention though, were the various photos of different people in military uniforms. One was a black male in his army dress uniform in front of the American flag. Another was a black male in his Navy dress blues. There was a picture of a white female in combat fatigues taken in front of the American flag. A picture of two black women, one wearing work and the other wearing dress whites taken in front of a naval ship. Another photo was of an Asian, possibly a Filipino male in an Air Force uniform. There were two pictures of two white males in their Marine dress uniforms, once again depicted in front of the American flag. There were several pictures of males in fatigues, some taken at Camp Pendleton, Camp Lejeune, Kaneohe Marine Corps Air Station, as well as Fort Bragg, Fort Drum, Fort Hood, and even Fort Hamilton. Several pictures of various naval vessels adorned the walls. A picture of the current President also took up space on the wall, as well as a picture of Dr. Martin Luther King Jr.

Preacher laughed to himself at the caption someone with the initials 'D.T.' wrote and placed under that picture. It read; "To Tristian: it's good to be the KING!" Preacher and Shamel felt very relaxed, and it showed.

"Can I offer you gentlemen some refreshments? Coffee, soda?" Tristian asked, as he gestured for Preacher and Shamel to have a seat in either of the two chairs.

"I'll have a Coke." Preacher enthusiastically answered.

"Ginger ale for me." Shamel answered.

"Think I'll have an ale too." Zachary said.

"Ok," Tristian replied, as he pressed the intercom button on his phone. "Ms. Kennedy?"

"Yes?"

"Two Ales, a regular and a Diet Coke please."

"Right away." the administrative assistant answered.

Agent King sat in the chair behind the desk, while agent Elvis stood off to the side behind him. "As I was explaining to you earlier Preacher, we had a major bust occur at one of our bases in Virginia. Some sailors were caught in a sweep. One in particular, 'Vicar Avaminx' who's an American citizen but was born in Russia was detained with the most circumstantial evidence."

"We suspect he may have been the fall guy for this drug cartel. Whether he was or not, he implicated himself and sparked our investigation to come north." Agent Elvis added.

"I take it he did himself a favor by trying to cut a deal." Preacher stated.

"Not really. Under article 112a of the UCMJ he was given 150 years of hard labor at USP Leavenworth." Tristian replied.

Preacher and Shamel both made faces, with Preacher exclaiming 'Wow!'

"Mind you, this guy is from DC. I feel for his relatives in a way, because he could've just given up whoever it is he's protecting, and not gotten such a raw deal. All he said was, 'My life is over, but I'm not going to do that to my family.'- whatever he meant by that."

"You say that he wrote a confession, but didn't give up the person or persons he worked for?" Shamel asked puzzled.

"Yes. Most of the information we obtained from him centered on the location of this drug cartel. But he refused to tell us who the ringleader is. All we know is that it's a civilian. That makes this even more disturbing, because there is no telling how many other military members are wound up in this." Agent King stated. "Past drug busts always ended up being small, close-knit operations, sometimes with fewer than 10 people involved. From what we've learned, this guy has military connections from Pensacola, probably up to Groton, CT."

"Probably?" Preacher asked.

"There's some major coup being planned. We don't know what is right now, but believe me when I say we're going to find out."

At that moment there was a gentle knock on the door.

"Come in." Tristian answered.

In walked the administrative assistant Ms. Kennedy with the sodas. Ms. Kennedy was a tall, svelte curvaceous woman with dirty blonde hair. She had on a dress that showed off her gorgeous legs. First, she walked over towards Preacher and inquired, "Was the Coke for you?" in a soft, pleasant voice.

"Yes." Preacher replied in an equally pleasant tone of voice.

She then placed a can of Coke, a napkin and a cup of ice on Tristian's desk near him.

"Thank you." Preacher said.

"You're welcome." she replied, repeating the same routine for Shamel, but with a can of ginger ale.

"Thank you." Shamel responded.

"You're welcome." she replied again.

She set down the other can of ginger ale, a napkin and a cup on the desk for Zachary.

"Thank you." Zachary said.

"You're welcome."she replied. Finally, she set down the napkin and cup, but also opened the can of Diet Coke and poured some into the cup of ice for Tristian.

"Thanks Fawn."

"Anytime, Tristian." she replied, as she turned and headed out of the office.

Preacher and Shamel watched her as she exited, then turned and nodded their heads while beaming at each other.

"What else can you tell us about this cartel?" Preacher asked as he opened his soda.

"One thing we know is that they're pretty large and violent. Part of their M.O. is to cut off a body part, usually a piece of the ear."

Shamel sat upright and restated, "They slice off the ear part of their victim?"

"Not just any victims. It's usually members who have had a falling out with the cartel. In 'Avaminx's' confession, he also made reference to a runner or transporter, but referred to him as brigadier. Our intelligence sources informed us that's Russian for soldier. So if this is the work of the Russian mafia, we've really got a problem on our hands." Agent King finished.

Shamel thought back for a moment about the body that Officer Valentine-Brown alerted him to. Just on a hunch, he decided to call and talk to Sequoia…

"Tristian, do you mind if I make a phone call? In fact I can do it right here in your office."

"Sure, phone is all yours." Agent King replied.

Shamel dialed the number to his precinct. After two rings, someone picked up.

"NYPD-BLING division. Detective Zapata speaking. How may I help you?"

"Angel! The hell you doing there this time of day?" Shamel chided.

"Everybody needs some money - and overtime…" Angel replied in singsong.

"You sure it's not a mandation?"

"All free will! Gotta save up for that trip to the Dominican Republic!"

"I feel you! Anyway, where's my partner at?"

"Hold on." Angel placed the phone on hold, and went to call Sequoia who was shooting the breeze with Lavender. "Quoia!" Angel yelled out.

"Si', Papi?" Sequoia gaily responded.

Gesturing with his hand, Angel made a phone handset and said "Llame!"

Sequoia nodded her head in acknowledgment, then turned to Lavender and said, "Talk to you later girl!" as she went to retrieve her call.

"Narcotics division. Detective Charms speaking."

"Sequoia! What's good?"

"Oh, is this the partner that abandoned me?" Sequoia replied sarcastically. "Your ears must be burning, because I was just talking about you! How's it going?"

"Things are okay. But would you believe I'm working? Helping my brother out with something. Have a question. Did the unit get a hit on a victim, who may possibly have been a drug runner?"

"Give me a basic description, Sha."

"I'll do better than that. Going to send you a pic right now."

"Ok."

Shamel pulled out his cell phone, and sent the pic of 'Yuri' he had taken to her. There was a brief pause, and then Sequoia said, "Damn, Sha. You must be psychic! Homicide called with some information for us on this body. Just so happens I have his file right here in my hand."

"Great! Hold on just a moment, Quoia."

Shamel then turned to agents King and Elvis and asked, "Did the guy who confessed give you a description of this brigadier?"

"White male, 20's, and Russian. If that fits the description of the person in your phone you just sent, would you mind beaming it to me? It appears we have the same model." Tristian respectfully requested from Shamel.

"Could you beam me that photo also? Looks like we all have the same phone!" Zachary stated.

"I feel so left out!" Preacher joked.

Shamel quickly beamed the photo to both agents, then turned his attention back to Sequoia.

"Hit me." Shamel said to her.

"The young male you're referring to is 'Yuri Blog' - like a blog. Terrible last name too if I may say so. Resident of DC, but also had a Virginia address. We got it from Homicide, because this guy had a lot of priors for drug possession."

"So did *Richard…*" - Shamel joshed.

"I will give you *a supervision* on your wack jokes later." Sequoia scolded. "Where are you calling from? I know it's Washington DC from the caller ID, but are you at their police precinct?"

"I'm actually with Naval Criminal Investigative Service. Seems like they have a hand in this investigation as well."

"Well, I hope this helps. And I also hope you'll be bringing your butt back to New York soon, playa. Leaving me to bust all these drug gangs by myself." Sequoia kidded.

"I'll be back soon enough."

"Ok. Don't make me cross the 'Delaware' to come get you!"

"Thanks, Quoia! Holla later."

"Bye, Sha!"

"Bye."

Shamel turned his attention back to Tristian and asked, "Does the name 'Yuri Blog' raise any eyebrows?"

"I believe we did come across that name, but we would have to dig a little deeper to verify." Agent Elvis said. "If anything, we hope to develop some more leads once most of the naval vessels return to Norfolk. Right now with everyone being in New York for 'Fleet Week', we haven't had much success in obtaining any information at all."

"Earlier, you mentioned that some major takeover was being planned. You don't suppose it has anything to do with 'Fleet Week', do you? Shamel asked.

Tristian, Zachary, and Preacher all looked at Shamel in astonishment.

"That's a good question! Do you know something we don't?" Tristian asked.

"Not at all. But this 'Yuri' kid was Russian. 'Avaminx' is Russian,-"

"And that guy at the safehouse I went to on a raid with Lieut. Merriweather is Russian!" Preacher butted in. "Looks like a conspiracy to me, but how does the navy figure in?"

"I'm scared to even come up with a theory. We'll just have to stay vigilant in these coming days to see what else transpires." Tristian answered.

At that point, he arose from behind his desk and walked around to the front.

"Preacher, Shamel, it was a pleasure meeting you both. On behalf of NCIS, I thank you for your time. Unfortunately, Zachary and I have to head over to Bolling AFB now, but we will have someone from the motor pool take you back."

"It was a pleasure meeting you as well." Preacher said, extending his hand to shake.

All four men shook hands. Tristian and Zachary then reached into their wallets, and pulled out two business cards each.

"Our direct numbers, as well as our cell phones. Please don't hesitate to call either one of us if you come across any information that you feel will be of benefit." Tristian encouraged. "In fact, we'd rather have a little bit of Intel, than a lot of *no tell*!"

"That's almost the same thing I say!" Shamel exclaimed.

"Glad to know we've got things in common!" Zachary cheered.

Each agent then handed Preacher and Shamel a card, which they both quickly looked at before putting into their own wallets.

"I'll have Ms. Kennedy arrange the pickup. Take care; hope to speak to you again soon." Tristian said.

"Likewise. Take care." Preacher replied, as Shamel nodded his head in acknowledgment.

Both Preacher and Shamel exited the office. As they walked by Ms. Kennedy's desk, they were going to say goodbye when she beat them to the punch. Smiling broadly and waving, Ms. Kennedy said, "Take care! Have a good day!"

"You too! Bye!" Preacher and Shamel both replied, as they continued to head towards the motor pool.

"Nice guys!" Shamel said to Preacher.

"Yeah. Nice secretary too!" Preacher replied.

They snickered amongst themselves as they arrived at the motor pool, where a transport vehicle was already waiting to take them back to VA.

Chapter Twenty-nine

The Baltimore-Washington Parkway (also known as Route 50) connects Baltimore Maryland from I-95 to Washington DC. It's a good alternative to I-95 in terms of both traffic and time. Unlike I-95, the Parkway is 29 miles of scenic highway with grassy terrain lined with trees almost its entire length. Patrolled by the US Park Police, it is this terrain which helps camouflage the police in their detection of speeders. One such patrol vehicle just made a U-turn onto the grassy terrain and was perpendicular to traffic headed towards DC. Like a spider waiting for prey to land on its web, the patrol vehicle sat still; ready to pounce on the first violator it caught on radar…

Seryoga was headed back to DC, after his errand in Baltimore. He was on the phone with Mstislab who was questioning him about the task. As usual, Seryoga had delegated the job to a brigadier, but pretended that he carried it out as per Mstislab's orders…

"So how did it go?" Mstislab asked.

"It was shot of vodka all the way!" Seryoga falsely boasted.

"I see. And I'm supposed to believe that you actually killed him like I ordered you to?"

"Yes Mstislab! You would have been so proud of me!"

"I can still be proud of you, when I see an earlobe. You did take an earlobe, did you not?"

Seryoga was trying to keep from being caught in a lie. He became nervous, and got a little heavy on his right foot…

"It was done, Mstislab!"

"So you say, but did <u>you</u> do it? It's not the question of it being carried out, but rather the issue that you disobey my direct orders! Remember our chat at American University? Can you fathom why I liken this 'family' to the 'Corleones'? What is it about loyalty you don't understand?"

"I could ask you the same question Mstislab. It's like you're trying to push me out with Stefan."

"You haven't been on top of things lately like I need you to be, Seryoga! You will always be my right hand man. But I need you to be more diligent and do what is expected of you. That includes carrying out execution orders. Things are only going to get more brutal, and I need to be certain that you will not punk out on me, Stefan."

"Uh, Mstislab-"

"I mean Seryoga!"

Mstislab corrected himself, but it was too little too late for Seryoga's psyche. Mstislab agitated Seryoga so much by calling him the wrong name; he wasn't paying attention to traffic or road conditions. The brake lights of two vehicles ahead of him came on, and they slowed down drastically. Seryoga was doing about 90 mph when he passed both of those cars – and streamlined himself right into the radar's Line of Site of the US Park Patrol vehicle on the median. The officer on radar patrol locked in Seryoga's speed, and pulled off the median into Seryoga's lane, accelerating to catch up to him. Seryoga was still trying to defend himself to Mstislab, and didn't notice he was being pulled over. This was a Dodge Charger, and Seryoga was in his Lexus. But Mstislab is the one who made a decision for him…

"You're headed back to the safehouse now, right?"

"Yes."

"Thomas is going to have six other guys who weren't going to be in New York meet you there. They'll help you finish packing up what's left. No evidence means no indictments."

"I want to be back in your good graces, Mstislab. But you have to- Oh *bog*!"

"What? Ready to confess your disloyalty to me?" Mstislab demanded.

"No! I'm being pulled over!"

"No the hell you're not! You still have everything in the car?"

"Of course!"

"Then I don't care how you do it, but you need to ditch that cop!"

"But Mstislab-"

"DON'T STOP! When I hear from you later, it had better be from New York, and not a Maryland jail!"

Mstislab abruptly hung up on Seryoga. By now the police cruiser had caught up to the Lexus and Seryoga had slowed significantly. It was just a matter of Seryoga obeying the law or following orders. He chose the latter. Seryoga pulled onto the shoulder with the patrol vehicle on his bumper, and came to a rolling stop, but left his foot on the brake. As soon as the officer came out of his vehicle, Seryoga put his foot back on the accelerator and floored it! The surprised officer immediately jumped back into his patrol car, and took off after Seryoga with emergency lights and siren. He also got on his radio for backup.

"This is Cpl. Newton with the US Park Patrol. I've got a felony evasive speed violator, headed southbound on 50. Vehicle is a black Lexus sport sedan. License plate, District of Columbia – **R**omeo, **U**niform, **S**ierra, **H**otel – **N**ovember. One male occupant. Be advised, high-speed pursuit now in progress."

"This is Cpl. Milner with the US Park Police. I'm heading towards the Greenbelt entrance now to render assistance."

There weren't many cars on the Parkway, but at the high rate of speed that Seryoga and the patrolman were going, they still had to precariously dodge around other vehicles. Seryoga was flashing his high beams and beeping his horn. At one point, he almost lost control of his vehicle as he dangerously shot between two cars occupying each lane, then dipped around a bus, nearly colliding with another vehicle in the process of switching lanes. The other patrol vehicle was just entering the Greenbelt entrance when Seryoga shot past. Taking the lead ahead of Cpl. Newton, he joined the chase which was nearing the end of the Parkway. Seryoga grew desperate. He now wished he had defied Mstislab and simply pulled over. But there was no turning back at this point. He needed a way out. Unfortunately at the expense of someone else, he found it. A woman driving a Lincoln Navigator was just a few feet ahead of the chase. Seryoga had a good quarter-mile lead on both patrol cars. That was all he needed to wreak havoc. Depressing the pedal all the way to the floor, Seryoga shot around in front of the Navigator. He then gripped the steering wheel tightly, and slammed on his brakes. The woman in the Navigator was so surprised at the impending collision; she immediately slammed on her brakes and swerved. The abrupt maneuver caused the Navigator to tilt and flip onto its side. Seryoga immediately hit the gas again, and screeched off. The first patrol car that was chasing after Seryoga couldn't stop in time to avoid colliding with the now flipped over Navigator. The front of the patrol car which had a bumper basher attached, struck the gas tank of the Navigator and punctured it, causing fuel to spill out onto the roadway. The force of the impact sent both vehicles sliding at least another 50 feet, before that Navigator struck the concrete divider, finally halting its momentum. The trail of spilled fuel followed the collision to its finish. Vehicles headed northbound on route 50 back towards Baltimore were slowing to witness the accident, as drivers began to rubberneck. Cpl. Newton in the second patrol vehicle skidded to a stop, and got out to assist both Cpl. Milner and the woman in the Navigator. Seryoga had stopped as well. He got out of the Lexus at the end of the Parkway just before it turned into local streets to witness the end result of his destructive action. The front of Cpl. Milner's police cruiser was smoldering from under the hood. Smoke was noticeably entering the passenger compartment. Cpl. Newton knew he had to act fast. He didn't have an extinguisher, so he ran over to the patrol car and assisted Cpl. Milner out. He then ran over to the Navigator and yelled out to the woman, "I'm going to get you out!"

"My kids," the woman's barely audible, muffled voice replied.

"What?"

"My kids. Please save my kids."

Undoubtedly, the vehicle's airbags help save the woman, and the two small children who were in the second row seat. Cpl. Milner was dazed, but he tried steadying himself to assist. Cpl. Newton crawled through the shattered rear window of the Navigator, over the third row seat to both kids in the second row seat. One child, a girl was unconscious. The other a boy, was slightly injured and crying. Fortunately they were seated in the middle and right seats, instead of directly behind the mother. Cpl. Newton undid the seatbelt of the boy first, and was able to hand him off to Cpl. Milner. Because the girl was unconscious, she was more cumbersome to deal with, but Cpl. Newton managed to unlatch her seatbelt as well, and carry her out. A third US Park Patrol vehicle pulled up, and the female officer got out to assist. Cpl. Newton handed the girl off to the third officer, then went to assist the driver. The driver must have felt or known that she wouldn't make it out of the vehicle however. Looking up at Cpl. Newton through her damaged windshield, she simply said, "Please tell my kids, mommy will always love them."

Now flames were highly visible as they shot out from under the hood and through the front grill of the police cruiser. "**Corporal Newton, it's going to explode!**" the third officer yelled at Corporal Newton, grabbing and pulling him over the concrete divider. As gas vapors in the air were igniting, the fire finally made contact with the ruptured fuel tank. In less time than it takes for a match to light, the entire tank exploded into an orange fireball, engulfing the Navigator, as well as the front end of the police cruiser. Seryoga decided he had seen enough. Getting back into the Lexus, he slowly drove away down New York Avenue and headed on to the safehouse.

Chapter Thirty

Preacher and Shamel had just returned to the precinct when they heard the police radio on the citywide frequency at the switchboard spew out the information on the accident.

"All units in the vicinity of route 50 ending southbound, accident with injuries, vehicles on fire, US Park patrol units already on scene."

"Sounds interesting! Wanna head over there?" Preacher said to Shamel.

"Sure! Maybe we can help in some way."

Preacher and Shamel got into the Jeep. With dazzle lights and siren, Preacher began to maneuver through the downtown traffic. He did not want to get stuck on Pennsylvania Avenue, so he made his way over to Massachusetts Avenue instead and took it until he could get onto New York Ave. When they arrived, the scene looked like a TV news segment out of the Middle East. DC Fire and EMS had already put out the vehicle fires, but were still hosing them down to cool them. Sand had been spread on the roadway where the spill occurred. A tow truck and a flatbed were both on standby to take the vehicles away. Other local police units from DC had arrived on the scene to aid in the accident. Two ambulances were off to the side. Preacher and Shamel noticed a group of officers including the US Park police near one of the ambulances and decided to approach them. With their shields in view, both Preacher and Shamel walked up to the group…

"Hey guys, what happened here?" Preacher asked.

Cpl. Newton spoke up; "This was a high-speed chase that ended with a woman losing her life. That big sport-utility vehicle over there? The guy I was after deliberately caused it to go out of control. The other US Park officer who was assisting me couldn't stop in time to avoid hitting it. We did manage to save two kids who are already in route to the hospital, but with the resulting fire, we couldn't rescue the woman."

At that moment, rescue workers carrying a body bag appeared. They gently placed the body bag on a waiting stretcher and strapped it in, then proceeded to place the stretcher into one of the ambulances.

"That is the remains of the woman." Cpl. Newton said apologetically.

A second stretcher appeared with Cpl. Milner strapped to it. Preacher and Shamel looked on sympathetically.

"Corporal Newton!" the female trooper who initially arrived on the scene called out.

"Yes, Trooper Band?"

"I have an address on that vehicle. It's registered to a 99 Sydney Terrace in the southeast part of DC."

Preacher's jaw dropped open.

"That's the same address we raided!" he exclaimed to Shamel. "Corporal, I know you have the situation under control here." He then turned to one of the DC officers and said, "Somebody get Lieut. Merriweather on the *horn*. Tell him we've got a level three priority mobilization at 99 Sidney Terrace! Come on, Sha!"

Shamel ran behind Preacher and jumped into the passenger side of the Jeep. Preacher quickly turned around and headed towards the southeast part of Washington, DC. He had no idea of what they were up against exactly, but he knew he couldn't stand by with that information and not help take action against the person responsible for the parkway carnage. Preacher also knew that if the car was registered to a known drug location, Metropolitan PD would need all the help they could get. That's when Preacher got on his cell phone and called the chief.

"This is Chief Fortson. What's going on, Preacher?"

"Chief, I know you heard about this accident on the citywide frequency. Could you have D.E.T.E.R. mobilize at 99 Sidney Terrace in 'the district'? DC Metro is going to need assistance!"

"You're second in command. Just be careful!"

"Always, chief! Thanks!"

Chapter Thirty-one

As Preacher and Shamel pulled up, Lieut. Merriweather had just arrived himself. An entire phalanx of heavily armed police was on standby. The street on both ends had been cordoned off. Sharpshooters were positioned along rooftops. Two K-9 units were also on standby, and just as a safety measure, the bomb squad was called in. Lieut. Merriweather nodded to Preacher and commented, "You sure know how to stir up an afternoon!"

"Major, this is my twin brother, detective Shamel Haynes, NYPD."

"Welcome to DC, even if there is a shootout!" Lieut. Merriweather quipped, as he quickly shook Shamel's hand. He then went into the trunk of his patrol car, and pulled out two bulletproof vests. He handed one each to Preacher and Shamel.

"I always carry extras just in case. But what made you call this level three, Preacher?"

"Cause and effect! Turns out the guy who caused the smashup on the Baltimore-Washington Parkway lives here!" Preacher replied.

The Lexus was parked a few doors down. It had already been seized by the Metropolitan police, who intended to tow it after the scene was secure. The Lieut. quickly hustled over to look at the car, then came back with a malicious smirk on his face.

"RUSH-N, huh? This is the break we've been waiting for! Good attention to detail, Preacher!"

"Preacher, do you need my team to do the entry?" A female lieutenant from D.E.T.E.R. approached and asked Preacher, while nodding and acknowledging 'Hello' to lieutenant Merriweather and Shamel.

"No, Lieutenant Apache. MPD has jurisdiction. We're just here to back them up, and since I'm not officially on duty, it's your call whether to engage or not. Hopefully this won't turn into a standoff."

Lieutenant Apache nodded her head again in acceptance as she went back to her staging position. Lieutenant Merriweather then turned and said aloud for all of the officers to hear, "All right! Use every precaution! We're going in!"

First, officers armed with machine guns entered the brownstone, followed by two officers with the battering ram this time. Behind them were Lieut. Merriweather, Preacher and Shamel, who were followed by more officers with machine guns. Everyone stood against the walls, while the officers with the battering ram stood at the ready.

"On my count. 3-2-1-GO!" Lieut. Merriweather yelled.

The officers with the battering ram charged full speed. With one loud bang, the door slammed open and the entire squad of officers poured in.

"MPD! EVERYBODY FREEZE!"

"POLICE RAID!" one of the occupants in the apartment shouted. He was immediately immobilized; thrown down to the floor and cuffed with a zip-tie. Other occupants were also quickly apprehended and cuffed where they stood or sat. In all six people were arrested, but there was no sign of Seryoga. This time, unlike the first raid, evidence was in plain view. There were kilos of cocaine lying on the coffee table waiting to be cut and distributed, alongside a scale. There were plastic baggies of Ecstasy pills. Four of the detainees had firearms on them. An AR 15 assault rifle and Mac-10 submachine gun were on the floor near the sofa. But one of the biggest pieces of damning evidence yet, was the duffel bag full of cash under the coffee table.

"I need a full room by room search of these premises for other offenders." Lieut. Merriweather ordered his officers.

Preacher and Shamel decided to assist. With his gun drawn, Preacher entered the bathroom. He turned on the light and quickly glanced at the tub. Not seeing anything amiss, he was about to walk out of the room when he pushed back on the door and heard a grunt. Stepping all the way into the bathroom, he swung the door closed - and stood face-to-face with Seryoga. Seryoga had a gun pointed right at Preacher, who in turn had his gun pointed right at Seryoga.

“Surely you didn’t think you were going to just walk out of here?” Preacher said to Seryoga.

“Maybe. But a hostage can improve my chances!” Seryoga replied, nervously.

“A HOSTAGE!” Preacher yelled out, hoping one of the other officers would hear him. “Considering we both have guns pointed at each other, who do you think is going to win?”

“Preacher!” Shamel yelled through the door.

“Don’t come in, Shamel! I’ve got a bit of a situation right now!” Preacher then calmly said to Seryoga, “I’m protected, you’re not.”

Realizing that Preacher was wearing a vest, Seryoga then raised his arm towards Preacher’s head. All the while he was trembling, which made Preacher very uncomfortable. Though Preacher knew what he was doing, he loved taking risks. This time, he slowly holstered his weapon, then raised both of his hands up towards his chest as he calmly said to Seryoga, “You’re scared. I don’t think you have the guts to pull that trigger.”

"I just want out!" Seryoga replied, his voice cracking.

"We can talk about this, but not with your gun pointed at me."

"Preacher! What's going on in there?" Shamel yelled again.

"This guy's got a gun on me!" Preacher yelled back.

On that, Shamel burst through the door. At the same time, Preacher ducked and lunged for Seryoga's arm. The gun in Seryoga's hand went off once, with the bullet lodging in the ceiling. Preacher and Shamel wrestled Seryoga to the floor. The gunshot immediately brought the other officers in the apartment to the bathroom, but by that time Seryoga had been subdued.

"I ought to break your wrist, but I think I'll just put your cuffs on real tight!" Preacher snarled at Seryoga.

Lieut. Merriweather pushed through the small crowd of officers and asked Preacher, "Are you ok? Are you shot?"

"I'm fine. My ears are ringing a bit, but I'll live!"

Preacher and Shamel brought Seryoga back out into the living room, and made him kneel on the floor next to the other six suspects. Six of the officers were checking the ID's of each one. One of the cops then yelled out, "Lieut.! We've got two guys here that are military!"

"We'll get them all back to the precinct for processing and interrogating. The military police have to be notified for those two."

"Hey Major? Do you mind if Shamel and I talked to this one? I think he has some real special things to tell us!" Preacher said, grabbing Seryoga by his shoulder.

"You're more than welcome to. Sergeant, please see to it that this apartment is properly secured. Good work all. Let's head to base."

Lieut. Merriweather headed out of the apartment, followed by the officers escorting each suspect. Preacher and Shamel led Seryoga out, with Shamel escorting him to a waiting police cruiser, while Preacher went to get his Jeep. Several officers began to seal off the area with yellow crime scene tape as the vehicles drove away to the Metropolitan police precinct to complete processing of the captured suspects.

Chapter Thirty-two

At the precinct, Lieut. Merriweather led in the officers with the suspects to the arrest room. Preacher asked Lieut. Merriweather for an empty interrogation room, which he and Shamel then led Seryoga to. Handcuffing one of Seryoga's wrists to the table, Preacher and Shamel then began to interview him.

"So you like pointing guns at cops. Am I going out on a limb here when I ask if you're part of the Russian mafia?" Shamel asked Seryoga.

"What difference does it make to you? You're just a cop. Me? I'm part of a large family that you'll never be able to control!" Seryoga replied.

"Well let me tell you an FYI. I'm from New York. I am part of the most elite narcotics unit in the state."

"And I'm with the best narcotics unit in VA" Preacher threw in.

"In any case, taking you and your *family* down is all in a day's work for us. Make it easy on yourself. Turn your boss over. Cut a deal. Because if you don't do it now, when we start making more arrests, you won't be able to talk your way out of a thing." Shamel informed him,

"Do what you want, I'm not talking." Seryoga defiantly declared.

"Something has to give. What can we do to make this guy comply with us?" Preacher asked.

"I don't know. Cut off his ear?" Shamel joked.

That joke however would prove to be exactly what the twins needed. For though he made the comment in jest, the look of horror on Seryoga's face was concerning. Seryoga had thought that the twins were just some dirty cops that Mstislab put on his payroll.

"Can we make this go away? I'm just a soldier myself. I follow orders and do what I'm told."

"Who told you to run from that US Park Patrol vehicle, and cause that accident?" Preacher rebuked.

"That was an unintended consequence. I would have stopped, but he might have confiscated all the money including what was set aside for you guys. I had to put a gun in some kid's face and make him understand, he was going to wind up on a slab for not having the correct amount already split. Forget what you saw in the house. We were going to transfer everything into an armored van."

Shamel felt a knot form in his stomach. His mind flashed back to the day he and Preacher were kids and the older teen boy pulled a gun out on them. It was vivid. All he could see was the barrel of the gun pointing right at him, and then he saw the casket of his father. He saw the casket being lowered into the ground. He heard the gunshot – then Shamel snapped. Pulling his gun out of its holster, Shamel cocked the hammer back, and pointed it at Seryoga's head.

"You guys cut me loose, I will ensure you get your cu-...What are you doing?" Seryoga abruptly remarked in a very jittery voice to Shamel.

"Shamel, what are you doing?" Preacher asked very concerned.

"This bastard! This guy is responsible for our father's death!" Shamel said, his voice choking with emotion.

"Shamel, dad was killed in a botched robbery attempt."

"Don't you see, Preacher? They're all linked! These guys sell the drugs and weapons that the criminals need money for, so the criminals go and commit the crimes that make us suffer!"

Shamel pressed the barrel of his gun against Seryoga's forehead.

"How does it feel to have a gun against <u>your</u> skull? Not a good feeling, is it? ANSWER ME!"

"No, no, no, it isn't!" Seryoga replied, sounding terrified.

"Shamel," Preacher said, gently placing his hand on the barrel of Shamel's gun, and lowering it. "You don't want to be the one facing the judge. Go get some water. I'll handle this."

Reluctantly, Shamel finally released the hammer and put his firearm away, then left the room.

"Wow! That guy's got issues!" Seryoga said.

"Mmm. Well, if he has issues, then so do I. We're brothers from the same mother." Preacher said, as he walked behind Seryoga. He bent over and whispered into Seryoga's ear, "I know people, who know people." He then stood up, walked in front of Seryoga and said, "I know people, who know how to get rid of bodies. You're from the DC area. Can you tell me how many square miles the Potomac is? Not that it would matter to you, but I think it's interesting to know just how much water someone would have to search through, to find body parts. That is, if the Marine life hasn't totally consumed them all."

"I don't understand." Seryoga replied.

"Let me make you understand." Preacher bent down and looked Seryoga right in his eyes, then said, "Have you ever seen what's left of a body that's been sucked through the jet engine of an F/A-18 Hornet, or an F-14 Tomcat? Pretty nasty. Hospital corpsmen run themselves ragged cleaning up those remains. But when you're way out in the middle of the Atlantic Ocean, it's a lot easier to just toss the remains off the side of the ship for the sharks, like chum, you know." Preacher continued, as he stood up, "The Chesapeake

Bay Bridge isn't a bad alternative for disposing of bodies either. See, getting rid of you is going to be fun! Especially since were obviously not going to get any information from you anyway."

Shamel reentered the room. He appeared sedate now, but Preacher could tell he was still upset.

"Hey Sha. I was just telling this guy about missing persons."

Shamel immediately caught on. His face lit up, and he played along.

"You know, your arrest hasn't been processed yet, so you don't exist in the system. In fact, we can hold you up to 72 hours. Then somehow, you'll magically wind up at CIA headquarters, where after they're done interrogating you, you'll be jailed on petition of the Patriot Act!"

Upon that, Preacher pulled out his own weapon, and forcefully slammed the barrel into Seryoga's 'private'.

Seryoga winced in pain and yelled out, "This is police brutality!"

"Aw, no! This isn't brutality. You haven't seen brutality! This is called coercion!" Preacher replied, as he then took Seryoga's left earlobe, and placed it between the hammer of his gun and the well.

"**Arrugh!**" Seryoga yelled out in agony.

"Now this is what you'd call brutality! Scream all you want. No one can hear you. These rooms are soundproofed. I can release the pressure on your ear at any time, you know. All I have to do is squeeze the trigger."

"***Chyort!** (*Damn, Hell)"

"What? You're ready to make a report? I can't **EAR** you!"

"All right! All right! I'll talk! I'll tell you everything! I'm not even the one in charge!"

"Who is?" Preacher demanded.

"Mstislav! Mstislav Diviodich! Ow! My ear!"

Preacher finally released the hammer from Seryoga's earlobe, which he quickly began to rub.

Shamel stood back amazed! He said to Preacher, "Nice tactic!"

"For him, it beats getting beat!" Preacher replied.

At that moment, there was a knock on the door and Lieut. Merriweather popped in. "How's it going in here?"

"We have a name, Major. Mstislav Diviodich." Preacher answered.

"I'll see if I can pull a file on him. I'm pretty certain it's an entire ream of paper!" Lieut. Merriweather joked, before exiting the room.

"As for you, start talking!" Preacher bellowed at Seryoga, tossing a pen and pad in front of him.

Seryoga kept his word, and began telling Preacher and Shamel everything. He told of how the military got involved to help with the smuggling. Preacher and Shamel had been in the room with Seryoga for over 45 minutes, when Seryoga dropped the bombshell on them.

"This Mstislav guy. Where is he now?" Shamel asked.

Seryoga didn't answer right away.

"Hammer time!" Preacher yelled, as he reached for his gun again.

"No, wait!" Seryoga pleaded. "Look, I had time to think about all of this. I want to say that I'm sorry. After all he's put me through, I should have just told you from the start what the deal was."

"Go on." Preacher replied.

Seryoga sighed, then continued, "Mstislav's in New York right now. There's a big shipment of drugs - and guns that he's having transported up to Boston."

"How big are we talking?" Shamel asked.

"When I say big, to quote Mstislav, I'm talking Wooly Mammoth! It's so big of a deal; he's not even worried about DC right now."

"Why didn't you tell us this in the beginning?" Shamel angrily demanded.

"At the same time you guys were busy arresting me and the few remaining *family* members, Mstislav was already in New York, preparing to leave!"

"Preparing to leave?" Preacher asked.

"Yes. You're probably too late, because the drugs and weapons are already there! Mstislav used the Navy to ship all the weapons to New York, as well as other members bringing guns through the *iron pipeline*. Everyone was supposed to meet up at a central location where they would give the guns to one person who will complete the trip. That's how he kept track of what he had."

"Is that why DC operated the safehouse, sort as a hub? Shamel asked.

"That was part of it. He lived here too you know!"

"But he used the Navy to get the weapons to New York because of Fleet Week and the fact that all the ships were going to be there anyway?" Preacher inquired.

"Now you've got it! Mstislav made a lot of friends who were assigned to ships, and was able to transport just about anything undetected. We had the perfect courier."

"Preacher, let me talk to you outside the room." Shamel said.

After they stepped outside the room, Lieut. Merriweather came walking back up to Preacher with a file in his hand.

"Here it is. He goes by the alias, 'Slab'. Interesting tidbit, he doesn't have too many arrests on his record. Must've had other people doing his dirty work for him, considering how sizable the gang is. He was court martialed by the Russian Navy on a charge similar to that of article 133 of the UCMJ – conduct unbecoming an Officer. Interpol was tracking him, then he fell through the cracks. Figures he would come to my city and be a pain, like Capitol Hill doesn't have enough 'Pork Barrel' projects. This guy just adds the street version!"

"Thanks, Major." Preacher responded, taking the file from Lieut. Merriweather.

As he and Shamel watched the lieutenant walk off, Shamel then said to Preacher, "This sucks! If I had known, I could've had my unit try to intercept them!"

"How do you think I feel? Both of us were sitting on top of a major weapons cache operation, and didn't know a thing! This was not my idea of a vacation for either one of us! Now the streets are going to be flooded with more guns! The question is, what can we do about it?"

At that moment, who should walk through the front entrance of the precinct, but none other than Special agents King and Elvis. Lieut. Merriweather had notified them of the two military people arrested in the raid. Preacher and Shamel looked at each other and gleefully said, "Call in the Navy!"

Chapter Thirty-three

At first glance, it looks like part of the Presidential motorcade. The black Chevy Suburbans with the red and blue flashing lights were definitely federal agents. But this wasn't the President. It was NCIS agents headed to Andrews Air Force Base. Shamel and Preacher informed agents King and Elvis about all that occurred, as well as what was going down in New York. Shamel called his supervisor to inform and have him prepare B.L.I.N.G. for what was going to be the biggest raid since BLING's inception. Two other agencies, the DEA and Port Authority Police had been notified as well. The DEA was participating in the raid with BLING and NCIS. The Port Authority Police were instructed to watch the bridges and tunnels for any suspicious vehicles that might be transporting the additional weapons that Seryoga told Preacher and Shamel about. Once the convoy arrived at Andrews AFB, everyone quickly mobilized to board the government owned private jet that would take them to

New York. Shamel handed copies of Mstislav's file with his photo to agents King and Elvis.

"We'll land at Stewart International airport and head out from there!" Agent King said to everyone.

"The old airbase in upstate Newburgh? Too far! We'll never make it back to the city in time!" Shamel protested.

"Sir, what about the Marine Air Terminal at LaGuardia Airport?" the pilot said.

"I have a better alternative. Floyd Bennett Field. It's also one of our staging areas, and it's right in Brooklyn!" Shamel said.

"Ok! Floyd Bennett Field it is then! Zachary, inform the NYPD and the DEA of our destination and estimated arrival time. This Mstislav or 'slab guy' is going down!" Agent King replied.

The jet took off, headed for New York and Floyd Bennett Field. Everyone just hoped they would arrive before it was too late.

Chapter Thirty-four

Upon arrival at Floyd Bennett Field, nearly the entire BLING unit was present. Everyone greeted Shamel, Preacher, and the NCIS agents. Some members including Angel looked weary, as if they had been awoken out of a sound sleep. Everyone appeared anxious. The DEA along with the NYPD's Communications Division, Aviation unit, and ESU, which the commanding officer of BLING requested for backup considering the nature of this particular raid, joined the narcotics squad. In all, excluding the few uniformed officers who were assigned to BLING, there were over 80 law enforcers present. Just about everyone was heavily armed. Though most of the officers had flak jackets, every BLING detective was identified with the nylon outerwear that had silkscreen printing on it. On the front of the jackets in bold lettering was NYPD. The back had the letters B.L.I.N.G. going across from left to right, also in bold lettering.

Angel approached Preacher, mistaking him for Shamel. He engaged Preacher in the cultural handshake/hug combination, then said, "Couldn't you have called this thing around 12 midnight?"

"I know how much you like overtime, so I wanted to make sure you had your fair share!" Shamel said, as he walked up.

Angel looked at Shamel, then looked back at Preacher, then did a quick double take of both of them.

"I thought cloning was banned!" he kidded.

"Angel, this is my twin, Preacher." Shamel replied.

"Detective Haynes; Alexandria, Va. Police." Preacher said to Angel, shaking his hand again.

"Wish I had a twin. He would be here, and I would be at home sleep! However, it's a pleasure to meet you. I'll catch up to you guys again later."

"Ok, Angel." Shamel replied, as Angel walked off.

Shamel was then approached by Sequoia, joined with Viper and Lavender. Sequoia had Shamel's jacket in her hand, which she handed to him.

"Welcome back, even though this is some kind of entrance!"

"You're telling me! By the way Sequoia, Viper, Lavender, this is my twin brother, detective Preacher Haynes, Alexandria narcotics unit."

"Nice to meet you! So sorry it's under these conditions!" Sequoia answered.

"Hey, work is work!" Preacher replied.

Viper and Lavender shook Preacher's hand and greeted him as well.

"Sequoia, do you think we might have an extra jacket that will fit him?" Shamel asked.

"You know we all have our own jackets.But I'll see if the supervisor has one in his car."

Sequoia dashed off, while the rest of BLING and the other agencies continued to assemble. Moments later, Sequoia returned with a jacket in her hand. Preacher thanked her and put it on. It fits somewhat snug, but Preacher knew it was only temporary. By now, everyone was gathered.

The Officer In Charge (or OIC) who held the rank of Captain, called for attention…

"As you all know, this is not a drill. The possibility of heavy casualty loss is high. Today, we as New York's finest have the distinction of working alongside two other very fine agencies in their own right - The DEA and Naval Criminal Investigative Service. I caution every one of you. Do not be thrown off by the fact that we're going after members of our Armed Forces. Of course I don't have to explain this to NCIS and the DEA, but for those of you in the NYPD who may be prior or even current military members such as the National Guard or reserves, bear in mind that these are criminals, and not the ambassadors that are supposed to represent our country. Any questions?"

No one said a word. Then, Viper spoke aloud,

"God Bless America, time to *BLING*!"

There was a unanimous cheer.

"All right, 'Operation Empty Clip' is now underway!" the OIC shouted.

All of the BLING units were unmarked and low profile vehicles. Preacher rode with Shamel, as did Sequoia and Lavender. DEA agents had their own vehicles. All of the NCIS agents were being transported in a combination of vans and cars, courtesy of the NYPD. Aviation lifted off, and headed out. Finally, both ESU with their huge emergency truck and the Command Post vehicle came last behind the other vehicles. Because trucks and buses aren't allow on parkways, two unmarked vehicles with emergency lights and sirens escorted the ESU and CP vehicles to the Brooklyn Marine terminal via Flatbush to Atlantic Avenue. Everyone else headed to the Belt Parkway for the trip - and probable battle on the Brooklyn waterfront.

Chapter Thirty-five

The USS Minotaur is a naval supply ship. Its main function is to bring supplies and goods to other ships that are deployed. Because of its capability to carry cargo, it turned out to be the best ship for Mstislab's operation. The entire Pegasus Carrier Group headed to Brooklyn due to space and ease of maneuverability. The Minotaur itself was docked at Brooklyn Marine terminal one, while the Pegasus was docked a few piers away at terminal seven. All of the other ships in the group were across the river in Manhattan, taking part in the Fleet Week celebration. While on deck of the Minotaur, one of the ships Boatswain's Mates noticed an oil spill. He immediately contacted his superior.

"Excuse me, Petty Officer Trellis."

"Yes, what is it?"

"I noticed what appears to be an oil leak on the starboard side of the ship, towards the aft."

Petty Officer Trellis looked over the side for himself, then commented, "There's a lot of marine traffic in these shipping lanes. I don't believe that's from us, but you can monitor the situation and keep the Officer Of the Day informed. Let the DC's and HT's know as well." Petty Officer Trellis said, referring to the Damage Controlmen and Hull maintenance Technicians who were responsible for all damage and repairs there needed to be made to the vessel.

"Yes, Petty Officer Trellis." The Boatswain's Mate replied before carrying on with his other duties.

About this time, the NYPD Aviation unit was hovering overhead, providing surveillance for the ground units. While the ESU and Command Post vehicles had not arrived yet, the entire convoy of law enforcement from Floyd Bennett Field was making its way off the Brooklyn- Queens Expressway on to Atlantic Avenue. Everyone turned their emergency lights and siren off, as they approached the main gate of the BMT. The first vehicle to pull up was carrying the OIC and other supervisors.

"Police emergency! I need access to the entire terminal." the Captain said to the security guard.

"Yes sir!" the guard replied, as he opened the gate to let all the vehicles in.

Meanwhile, over at terminal four, Mstislab was pacing back and forth. He had chain-smoked about six cigarettes, and was working on his seventh when he finally spoke up.

"Where the hell are these guys? I'm going to kill them! All of them! I can't get in touch with Seryoga; he doesn't answer his cell phone. He better not had gotten caught by that cop he told me about! But where the hell are Jaska and Nunchaku?"

"Mstislab, did Seryoga tell them to take the Goethals-Verrazano Bridge combo?" Stefan asked.

"The go-what?" Mstislab responded.

"Exit 13 off the New Jersey Turnpike. The Goethals to the Verrazano Bridge. It would have put them right in Brooklyn and brought them right here from the Expressway. You were asleep this morning when I took that in."

"Indeed. But I think Seryoga told them to take the George Washington Bridge."

"Bad move." Stefan replied, shaking his head. "Maybe that's why they're taking so long. They'll have to go all the way downtown to the Manhattan Bridge, just to come back into Brooklyn. With it being rush-hour, there is no telling how long it will take! But if I may ask a dumb question, why don't you just call them?"

"Because **both** of those numb-nuts cell phones are dead! Jaska called me from that last rest stop on 95 in Maryland with a *calling card,* telling me this nonsense! I told him they better hit a 'Radio Shack' and get car chargers, but that was over three hours ago! I'm really annoyed with those two 'commies' right now!

"Mstislab, I only have liberty for 48 hours. We need to get going now." Thomas said.

"I agree, 'Slab'." Stefan said.

"But I need these guns!" Mstislab implored.

"Well, Mstislab, we did manage to acquire some firearms. I got in touch with Anatoly. He has contacts inside the Naval Weapons Station, and was able to come through for the *family*! I know that Jaska and

Nunchaku have the bulk of the automatic weapons, but at least we've got artillery if we need it." Thomas said.

"What type?" Mstislab asked.

"Good 'ol American muscle. We even managed to get some AK-47's, though they didn't come from the military."

"Here's what we can do. If Jaska and Nunchaku contact you while we're on the road, tell them to come up towards Boston. We can always wait for them in Todeowilde." Stefan reasoned.

"I hate that part of Rhode Island."

"Another thing, Mstislab. We need to get out of here, before anyone gets suspicious. All the drugs and weapons are off. But if we keep hanging around, both the MA's and civilian guards are going to start asking questions."

"Yeah. We almost had to do one of them early this morning while we were offloading. Lucky for him, he believed us when we said it was just general supplies." – another sailor that was part of the operation threw in.

Mstislab took a puff and blew the smoke out through his nostrils. He then said, "I'll give them ten more minutes. You guys know I like to have everything together! I can't have my Boston cr-" "Mstislab, you know they're already armed." Stefan challenged, cutting him off. "You just want these guns as a means of getting extra cash. I don't think that should be your main concern right now." Mstislab gave Stefan a stern look, but Stefan just apathetically shrugged his shoulders. "I'm telling you right. I wouldn't paint myself into a corner, and I don't want you to do the same. Trust my judgment. You didn't make me your new right-hand man for nothing."

"Ten more minutes, then we leave." Mstislab replied.

He threw down his half-smoked cigarette in disgust, and promptly lit up another one. By this time, the ESU and Command Post vehicles had arrived. The CP bus was stationed outside the terminal at the main gate to assist with radio communications for the ground units. The ESU truck was on standby on Atlantic Avenue, with its officers ready to spring into action if needed. Everyone actively involved in the operation assembled inside terminal one.

"We'll break down into eight groups of 10. I need one BLING detective from each group to act as team leader. The last group however will be under NCIS jurisdiction." the OIC said.

Tristan and Zachary both approached the OIC.

"That's the ship right there, the USS Minotaur. I'm going to have some of my agents' board it along with the ship's own security and some DEA agents to perform a thorough deck by deck search. We need to get in touch with the CO and XO to let them know what's going on." Tristan said.

"First, we need to shut the terminal down. No one gets in, and no one gets out." the OIC replied.

Shamel then approached the OIC and said, "Captain, I think we need to mix the groups to search for this Mstislav guy. We know what he looks like, but he has naval personnel with him and that may throw us off."

"I agree. I don't want any sailor who should be arrested feigning as if they're just an innocent bystander. They could always run back to their ship and act like they were never involved." Tristan said.

"Ok. I'll have the uniformed officers cover the gates. Be careful and good luck!" the OIC replied.

"Thank you." Shamel answered.

Shamel, Preacher, Tristan, Sequoia, Lavender, and five other hand-picked law enforcers comprised of two BLING detectives, one NCIS agent, and two DEA agents formed the first group. Viper, Angel, and a combination of other officers made up the second group. Zachary was leading the final team of the eight groups onto the Minotaur for the deck by deck search. The other seven groups fanned out inside the terminal to look for the weapons – and Mstislav, before they could make their way up to Boston. No one over in terminal four had any idea the police had arrived - but that was about to abruptly change.

Chapter Thirty-six

Thomas was very restless. Stefan began to grow impatient. Mstislab was cursing and muttering to himself under his breath. BLING and the other police agencies were conducting their search, terminal by terminal. The police aviation unit radioed to the command post vehicle about a group outside terminal four that didn't quite appear to be military or civilian employees. That information was relayed to Shamel's group who radioed back that they would investigate. From a distance, Shamel couldn't tell what anyone in the group looked like. Taking cover behind a forklift and some other heavy equipment in the yard, Shamel asked Sequoia if she had her binoculars on her. He took them and was able to confirm identification. Peering through the lenses, Shamel fixed his gaze right on Mstislav.

"I'll be damned! He's still here!" Shamel excitedly affirmed.

"That means the drugs and weapons are still here then!" Tristian also excitedly commented.

Shamel then got on the police radio.

"BLING Special Ops team one to CP; we have a visual confirmation of all suspects. Requesting backup at Marine terminal four."

"This is Viper, BLING Special Ops team two. We're on our way to assist!"

"I'm not trying to be a hero, but you don't believe we can take these guys ourselves?" Tristian asked Shamel.

"I'm just following the SOP (Standard Operation Procedure). Of course, if you think we can take ém, then I think we can take ém!"

"I think we can take ém!" Sequoia confidently stated in a low tone of voice.

"Me too!" Lavender backed.

Soon the entire team was letting their egos get the best of them. Shamel quickly quieted them down then said, "Well, let me ask my reflection." referring to Preacher. "What do you think we should do, *Shamel*?" Shamel queried Preacher.

"Well, *Preacher*, if I were you, I would follow my first mind and instincts." Preacher replied to Shamel, punching the palm of his left hand.

"It's settled!" replied Shamel.

"Don't do that too often, or you'll confuse everybody including yourselves!" Sequoia said to both of them.

Shamel got back on the radio and said, "BLING Special Ops team one moving in!" as everyone in his group cautiously approached the terminal. By now, Mstislav and the others had moved way inside the terminal towards the rear, and had no idea what was about to transpire.

Shamel's team managed to slip inside the terminal undetected. Taking cover behind shipping containers, they all listened intently to Mstislav's conversation.

"Mstislab," Stefan pleaded.

"Ok! All right! We're moving out. Thomas, you say the trucks are ready?"

"Been ready, Mstislab! Just waiting on you!" Thomas replied.

"Everything is here in the back. We covered the Hummer with tarp, so it would look like cargo." Stefan said.

"Ok. We'll take the Manhattan Bridge to the West Side Highway, then hop on 95 north. Do we need to gas up or anything?"

"All covered." Stefan answered.

Mstislab smiled. Finally, it seemed he was pleased. Mstislab looked at a row of trucks and asked, "How many of those trucks belong to us?"

"All three! We got a little worried, because we thought we would need a fourth!" Zalitokessi, another *family* member answered.

"We've got the weapons in the back of the first truck." Thomas added.

"Damn! Now that's what I'm talking about! Boston, here we come!" Mstislab hollered.

"Russian Mafia!" Thomas bellowed.

"M.A.D. for life, baby!" Stefan yelled, as he and Thomas uncovered the Hummer from under the tarp.

“We won’t have a problem getting out of this place will we?” Mstislab asked Thomas.

“Nah. They usually only check the trucks that are coming in, never going out. If anything, all I have to do is show my military ID, and say we’re all together, including you.”

Shamel figured now was the time to announce their presence. He whispered to the entire team, “On my count, 3-2-1- Go!”

Shamel and Tristian both stepped from behind the shipping container with their shields visibly displayed from around their necks, and holding automatic weapons. Shamel declared out loud, “**Mstislav! NYPD!**” and Tristian yelled, “**NCIS!**”

“**Chyort!**” Mstislav screamed, as he pulled out the Beretta 9mm from his waistband and began firing, making everyone scatter!

“**Take cover!**” Shamel yelled out to his team, as he ducked back behind the container and returned fire.

"Stefan! Get to the truck! Get the truck out of here!" Mstislav yelled as he kept firing and ducking to avoid being hit.

Stefan, Thomas, and Zalitokessi were thinking like Mstislav. The trucks were lined up side-by-side. They went into the back of the truck with the automatic weapons which were already loaded, picked up a weapon each, and began firing from in-between the trucks and around the sides.

"SHOTS FIRED IN TERMINAL FOUR! WE HAVE SHOTS FIRED IN TERMINAL FOUR!" Tristian yelled into his radio.

"Tell your boys to grab a truck, and let's get out of here!" Stefan shouted to Thomas.

"Yo! Get in the trucks!" Thomas yelled out, as he and Stefan kept firing. Thomas jumped off the back of the truck with a US military issue M-240 rifle in his hands and began spraying back and forth, trying to provide the necessary cover fire for the drivers to get behind the wheel. Zalitokessi fired off rounds from an AR-15 rifle as he advanced forward to the driver's side of the first truck. Even though Shamel, Tristian, and five of the other law enforcers had automatic weapons themselves, they realized they were being outgunned. Preacher, Sequoia and Lavender only had their service and back up weapons. The M-240 which could fire up to 1000 rounds per minute was proving to be Mstislav's juggernaut, and team one's worst adversary. At the moment, all of them were pinned in their positions. Lavender screamed out in anguish, as everybody in the team cowered on the ground, frozen by the fusillade.

Mstislav emptied his 9mm and yelled out to Thomas, "Throw me a rifle!"

"Thomas threw Mstislav his M-240, while Stefan threw Thomas an M-249 SAW rifle, then picked up an M-16A2 rifle for himself.

"Give everybody a rifle!" Mstislav yelled out again, as he continued to spray bullets from the M-240.

Like a professional basketball team practicing free throws from the foul line, all of the members of Mstislav's *family* in a row were able to quickly grab a rifle, and continue the perilous assault on Shamel's team.

"TEAM ONE UNDER HEAVY FIRE! WE NEED BACKUP NOW!" Shamel screamed into his radio.

"Trucks, now!" Thomas yelled over the din.

With many of the members still firing away, the three drivers finally managed to hightail it into the trucks, which had the keys already in their ignitions.

"Mstislab!" Stefan shouted.

"Just throw me another rifle! I'm getting the Hummer!" Mstislav yelled back.

Stefan threw Mstislav another firearm – an MP 5 submachine gun, before finally jumping off the back of the truck and closing the cargo door. Shamel knew if his team stayed in that battlefield like atmosphere, they risked losing their lives.

"FALL BACK! GET OUT!" Shamel yelled to his team. Everyone began to cautiously make their way out of the terminal, still under heavy fire. At the same time, all three trucks were being started up.

"Keep shooting! We'll blast our way out of here!" Thomas yelled out to the *family,* as he made his way to the driver's side of one of the trucks. "Move over, I'll drive!" he told the person behind the wheel.

Stefan ran around to the passenger side of the truck with the weapons and climbed in. The first truck to pull out was the one in the middle. Thomas in the last truck was the second one to pull out. Finally, Stefan and Zalitokessi's truck with the weapons began to follow behind the others. Everyone in Shamel's group made it out of the terminal except him and Preacher.

Preacher crawled over to Shamel while they were both still crouched on the ground and said, "We can't let him get away!"

"I don't intend to! As soon as he runs out of ammo, we'll corner his ass!" Shamel replied.

Mstislav was still firing off a salvo of rounds when the M-240 suddenly went quiet. Shamel and Preacher heard the familiar clicking of an empty firearm having its trigger pulled and knew they had to act right then and there.

"Get him!" Shamel yelled, as both he and Preacher were finally able to get up, and return fire. Mstislav himself was taking cover behind some shipping containers. He dropped the M-240, and began firing with the MP 5 submachine gun he had in his possession. But this time, the tables were going to be turned. As Shamel and Preacher cautiously advanced towards Mstislav's location, Mstislav made the critical error of stepping out from behind the shipping container in full view. Immediately taking combat positions, Shamel and Preacher continued firing, and managed to strike Mstislav in both of his legs. Mstislav yelled out in pain and collapsed, but still kept firing off rounds himself from the assault rifle. Meanwhile back outside, Viper and team two had reached the terminal just as all three trucks were making their way towards the gate. Team two along with the group from team one that made it outside, opened fire on the first truck, blowing out its tires and causing it to crash into a shipping container. Thomas in the second truck was determined not to be stopped. He was firing his assault rifle out of the window, and managed to strike at least two law enforcers. Thomas intended to ram through the gate near terminal four, but to his amazement, the gate was already open. He slammed on the accelerator and managed to burst through the opening - but was abruptly stopped by colliding into the enormous ESU truck, which came to assist at terminal four once the shooting began. Surrounded by a small army of heavily armed police wearing tactical gear, Thomas and the accomplice seated next to him had no choice but to surrender. Stefan seeing what had occurred, told Zalitokessi to head towards the main gate. Law enforcers opened fire on his truck as well, with Stefan returning fire much like Thomas had. Zalitokessi managed to turn the truck and was about to speed towards the main gate, when Tristian stepped out right in front of the vehicle.

"Run his ass over!" Stefan barked at Zalitokessi, who slammed his foot on the gas, giving the truck a lot of momentum.

Tristian bravely and boldly took aim with his weapon, and fired upon Zalitokessi. The shots found their mark, striking Zalitokessi center mass in his chest. He expended a few final breath sounds, then slumped over the steering wheel with his foot still on the gas pedal. Stefan panicked, and grabbed the steering wheel. He began turning it wildly, sending the truck spinning out of control. All of the law enforcers scrambled to avoid being struck. Stefan figured his best plan of escape now was to abandon the truck and make a run for it. With all of his might, he managed to steer the truck towards terminal three. Bracing for impact, Stefan allowed the truck to crash into the structure of the storage facility, where after that deafening sound of steel colliding with steel, the truck finally came to halt. Though he was a bit disoriented, Stefan managed to scramble out of the truck, and after firing off a few rounds in the direction of the law enforcers, ran into the terminal in an attempt to hide. The drama outside the terminal was over, but the law enforcers knew they had to find and subdue Stefan, as well as another *family* members who may have slipped through the cracks during the fracas.

"Spread out! I want him taken alive if possible, but dead if necessary!" Viper shouted to both teams.

Sequoia and Lavender stuck together, both entering exactly where Stefan had entered into the terminal. Viper, Angel, Tristian and the others all split up and headed in different directions within the terminal to look for him as well. Shamel and Preacher were still fighting their own battle with Mstislav, but it seemed they were finally getting the upper hand. Though injured, Mstislav still put up a valiant struggle. He began to roll over repeatedly, firing as he did so in an attempt to make it to the Hummer. Preacher finally emptied out his service firearm, and went to retrieve his backup weapon.

"I'm going in to take this bastard down!" he shouted to Shamel.

"I've got you covered!" Shamel yelled back, as he continued to fire sporadically.

Preacher was able to sneak in a bit closer to Mstislav's position, but Shamel began to feel very uncomfortable not being near his brother. As Shamel began to move in closer himself, that decision would prove to be a lifesaver. Mstislav managed to get near the Hummer, and pulled himself up. He winced in pain, but was finally able to get himself positioned to get in the SUV. Preacher had Mstislav in his *crosshairs* and decided that this was a now or never opportunity.

Just as Mstislav got in the Hummer and closed the door, Preacher yelled out,

"Freeze or I'll shoot!"

"Bite me, policeman!" Mstislav yelled out as he opened fire again from the submachine gun out of the driver's window.

Preacher immediately took cover behind some nearby cargo and squeezed the trigger on his firearm - but got nothing. He released the clip, slapped it back in and tried again. Nothing. "Shamel! My weapon's jammed!" Preacher yelled out in panic.

Mstislav was still firing away, when Shamel reached for his own backup weapon and yelled out to Preacher, "CATCH!"- tossing the .357 Magnum in the air. Preacher managed to catch it, and upon quickly getting it handled, stepped from behind his barrier and assumed the combat position letting off a barrage of shots, emptying the revolver. The powerful shells found their mark, as one of the bullets ripped through Mstislav's arm, forcing him to drop the submachine gun. Another bullet shot out the passenger rear window. Though the trajectory of the other two bullets missed altogether, the final shot actually grazed Mstislav's face, forcing him to lie back in the seat as a means of protection. Now it was quiet. Shamel ran over to Preacher and helped him up. He handed Preacher a speed reloader and asked,

"Do you think we got him?"

"I don't know." Preacher replied, as he discarded the empty shells out of the Magnum and reloaded it. "But thanks for saving my life!" he said to Shamel.

"Don't dump the 'Gatorade' just yet! If he's still alive, neither one of us may walk out of here under our own power!" Shamel replied breathlessly.

"Shame on you! Where's your optimism?" Preacher scolded.

Shamel looked towards the Hummer and said, "Hopefully, lying dead in that SUV!"

Back in terminal three, Viper was patrolling for Stefan. He came around a shipping container when a shot rang out, and he felt a burning sensation in his left arm. Viper jumped back behind the container and saw his arm bleeding from a bullet wound. Instead of carrying an automatic weapon like the other law enforcers, Viper had a Mossberg 500 Cruiser shotgun with a pistol grip. He decided the best defense was self-defense, and purposely stepped from behind the container again in full view of his assailant. Sure enough, it was another *family* member who had ran into terminal three to hide out when the commotion began. He took aim at Viper once more, but this time Viper did not give him the opportunity to fire. Viper let off a round from his shotgun. The blast caught the *family* member in the chest knocking him backwards, before he collapsed and lay motionless. Viper himself sat down, and got on his radio.

"This is a Viper from BLING Special Ops team two. Officer down. Requesting assistance in terminal three."

Viper listened as his radio churned out conversations from the CPV, supervisors, and other teams while he waited for help to arrive. Sequoia and Lavender on the other hand were hot on Stefan's trail. They both cautiously peered around containers, cargo and heavy equipment looking for him.

"Split up?" Lavender asked Sequoia.

"Sure. Just be careful!" Sequoia replied.

"You too!" Lavender responded.

But no sooner had they separated when Lavender heard a noise. Stefan had been lying flat on top of a container. He jumped down right behind Sequoia and was about to shoot her.

"SEQUOIA, BEHIND YOU!" Lavender screamed.

Sequoia barely had time to react, but fortunately Stefan had that assault rifle. First, she deliberately tossed her own firearm on the ground, which caught Stefan off guard. Using the length of the assault rifle to her advantage, Sequoia stepped to one side and grabbed the barrel with both hands, forcefully pulling Stefan towards her. Sequoia then took her left hand and delivered a powerful heel strike with her palm to the bridge of Stefan's nose, forcing him to relinquish his hold of the rifle. Sequoia then immediately grabbed the back of the rifle with the hand she used for the heel strike and rammed the butt of it into Stefan's abdomen. Finally, grabbing the rifle like a baseball bat, she clubbed Stefan with it, sending him crashing to the ground! As Stefan lay moaning in pain, Sequoia pulled out the clip from the rifle, and handed both to Lavender as she came running back up.

"Oh my God, Sequoia! I'm so sorry!" Lavender asserted.

"Don't be! If we hadn't split up, he probably would have shot both of us. In a sense, we saved each other!"

Sequoia reassured, as she retrieved her firearm. Pulling out a pair of handcuffs, Sequoia bent down to Stefan and said, "Next time you want to shoot a woman, just remember that SIZE DOES MATTER!"

She and Lavender could hardly contain themselves, as she put the cuffs on Stefan, read him his rights, and escorted him out of the terminal. All that remained was to secure Mstislav, and it was all over. But Mstislav was not dead. He also wasn't about to give up so easily. His hand just happened to touch the Glock that was lying on the floor in the back of the Hummer – the same Glock he had tossed back there when he took over the SUV from Yuri. Mstislav got a firm grip of the gun, and took a deep breath. He knew that trying to drive out would be futile, and he would have to find another means of escape, even if it meant swimming away. Preacher and Shamel slowly approached the Hummer. Shamel was going to open the door, and Preacher would, if necessary open fire. To their surprise, that wasn't going to happen. Without warning, Mstislav spilled out of the Hummer, firing rapidly and wildly at the both of them!

"TAKE COVER!" Shamel yelled to Preacher, pushing him out of the way, and diving to the ground himself.

Although Mstislav was injured, he managed to summon up enough strength to actually run as he fired. This time, neither Preacher nor Shamel got a chance to shoot back, which really angered Preacher.

"What the hell! Are there two of him as well? Where did he go? WHERE ARE YOU, MSTISLAV?" Preacher said aloud, as he went off alone.

"Hey Preach! Hold on!" Shamel yelled after him, as he was changing clips in the automatic weapon.

Mstislav was desperate to escape, but he knew that he had to conserve bullets. Putting the Glock in his waistband, he looked around for something else he could wield as a weapon. Upon seeing a medium length thin pipe, Mstislav picked it up, and stood silent behind a row of containers. Unfortunately, Preacher allowed his anger to blind him. He got careless and started rushing around corners. As soon as he rounded the container where Mstislav was hidden from view, Mstislav pounced, striking Preacher on the right arm. Preacher yelled out in pain and dropped the Magnum as he also fell to the ground. Mstislav swung again, but in his own rage, missed altogether, striking the container instead. However, that energy and vibration from the blow traveled back up the pipe to Mstislav's hands, making him let it slip and land near Preacher. In addition, the loud clang seemed to ring throughout the terminal. It definitely caught Shamel's attention, as he yelled out "PREACHER!" and rushed in the direction of the noise.

Mstislav had murder in his eyes. He wanted to kill Preacher, and Preacher could tell. Mstislav realized that Preacher had dropped the Magnum. But as he attempted to retrieve it to turn on Preacher, Preacher tripped him. Mstislav quickly scrambled to his feet to try again. But Preacher being closer to the pipe, picked the pipe up and lobbed it will all his might at Mstislav. The pipe found its mark on Mstislav's head, striking him on the left temple. Dazed and bleeding, Mstislav stumbled off. Now Shamel had reached the area. Seeing Preacher on the ground, Shamel helped him to his feet.

"Careful Sha! My arm! I don't think it's broke, but it hurts like a son of a bitch!" Preacher moaned.

"Where's Mstislav?" Shamel asked.

"He's tripping, literally! I hit him with that pipe and he ran off. This can't go on much longer. Not the way he's injured!"- Preacher gasped, as he finally regained possession of the Magnum.

"Come on. Let's get him before anyone else gets hurt!" Shamel persuaded.

Mstislav had made his way outside through the rear exit, towards the piers. He saw his potential means of escape, and approached, determined to succeed. A male couple was enjoying themselves and their luxury speedboat, as were most of the boaters participating in the Fleet Week festivities. Pulling out the Glock, Mstislav bellowed to them, "Out of the boat!"

In defiance, one of the males who happened to be smoking stood up and said, "Who died, and made you Queen?"

Mstislav shot him in the abdomen. The man let out a screech of pain as he dropped the cigarette, then stumbled and fell overboard.

His partner pleaded with Mstislav; "Take the boat! It's a tax write-off for us anyway!"

Upon that, he jumped in the water to try to help his companion out. Fortunately they both had life vests on. Preacher and Shamel came running out as fast as they could upon hearing the gunshot. Mstislav had already hopped into the boat and started it. He was detaching the moor lines when Shamel and Preacher together yelled at him, "**STOP!**"

"This is your final warning, Mstislav! Slob! Slab! Whatever your confused mother put on your birth certificate!" Shamel hollered.

"We'll both shoot!" Preacher shouted as well.

"Not if I shoot first!" Mstislav shouted back. He pulled the Glock out of his waistband again and squeezed off two rounds.

Preacher and Shamel were both poised in the combat position. They returned fire, striking Mstislav in the torso and upper part of his body. The shots knocked Mstislav back, causing him to slam the boat into gear. The boat took off, headed towards terminal one where the Minotaur was docked. Mstislav was a bit delirious. He started laughing at the belief that he had gotten away.

"I'll live! I'll get treated and still run things!" he thought to himself.

Mstislav sat up, and fired a shot into the air.

"*Do svidaniya (duh svee-dah-nee-ye - *Goodbye)! I'm alive! And I'm going to explode!" - he yelled back towards the pier where Preacher and Shamel were still standing. Mstislav didn't know just how correct he was. Picking up the cigarette his victim dropped, Mstislav took a drag on it, and then turned around - just in time to see the speedboat about to collide with the Minotaur. Mstislav let out a high-pitched shriek of terror and surprise, as the speedboat rammed into the side of the ship. The force knocked the cigarette out of Mstislav's hand into the water, which mixed with the oil causing a small explosion and fire. All of the personnel came over to the right side of the ship to witness the accident, at which point the ship sounded its alarm…

"General Quarters! All hands on deck! Emergency - Starboard side!" – wailed the Public Address system on the Minotaur.

Preacher and Shamel witnessed the entire event. They then turned towards each other, and rejoiced in the moment.

"Now I must admit, that's not quite the end I was expecting to this whole ordeal, but that end justifies '**The Mean'**!" Preacher chortled, making the quotation symbol with his fingers.

"Might as well be Christmas, *cause* it's a wrap! Makes life easier for the police Marine unit too! There goes one now!" Shamel happily sighed.

Now it was truly over. As the police Marine unit which wasn't part of the operation cruised over to the accident to investigate, Preacher and Shamel both went to assist the male couple that Mstislav boat-jacked. While things continued to calm down, all of the teams gathered back at terminal one, where both a triage and arrest-processing center had been established. As for the detainees, they were already separated into civilian and military prisoners. One of the Carrier Group's senior military officers, Rear Admiral Sum-Yam addressed the military prisoners. He was none too pleased at the task, but did so with the utmost military bearing.

"All of you, who have been arrested, are a disgrace to the U.S. Navy, the United States of America, and to every decent, honest member of our Armed Forces. Upon return to Norfolk, you will all immediately receive a 'Captain's Mast'. Until then, Master at Arms, take them away!"

All of the military members involved were whisked away to the ship's brig on the Pegasus.

"The civilians will all be going to the Brooklyn House of detention. No doubt that some of them will be doing federal time along with these military guys." the OIC said to Rear Admiral Sum-Yam.

"Nice work. It's too bad things had to end this way for the Navy. But I'm glad they were stopped before it got way out of hand." Rear Admiral Sum-Yam said to the entire group. "As for the rest of you sailors, carry on!"

A unanimous "Aye-aye Sir!" was heard, as the sailors who were not involved continued about with their daily routines.

EMS was busy treating all of the wounded officers, none of whom had life-threatening injuries. Even the man who Mstislav had shot was going to survive. All the bodies of the *family* members that were killed had been moved back into terminal four, out of view of the public and the media while both NCIS agents and BLING detectives attempted to identify who was who. Even Mstislav's remains had been recovered from the wreckage of the speedboat, and were lying inside a body bag within the terminal, pending positive identification. Viper was about to be spirited away to the hospital, as was Preacher. But Shamel was nowhere to be found.

"Hey, has anyone seen my twin brother, Shamel?" Preacher yelled out.

"Was he hurt?"

"No."

"Maybe he just went on to the hospital ahead of us anyway. We're all going to 'Bellevue'."- Viper finished saying, before he was popped into the back of an ambulance. Preacher was curious, but figured Shamel would definitely catch up to him later. Shamel didn't tell anyone, but he decided to run back to the precinct to freshen up. He asked two uniformed officers from his precinct if they would take him back uptown, to which they agreed. After he was dropped off, Shamel went and showered, changed clothes, then got into his own car and headed downtown to 'Bellevue' with emergency lights and siren hoping no one had missed him too much, or at all.

Chapter Thirty-seven

At Bellevue Hospital Center, it seemed like more police were present there than at the Brooklyn Marine terminal. The Police Commissioner and other top brass as well as the Mayor had stopped by to congratulate and wish all the law enforcers a speedy recovery. Preacher had been seen and discharged quickly for blunt trauma injury. Though his arm was still smarting from the blow he suffered at the hands of Mstislav, he declined the use of a sling, opting to hold ice on the bruise instead. The law enforcers who had been shot were being admitted for observation, and Viper was having his wound cleansed and dressed. While the media was there, a brief statement was given by the police spokesperson of the condition of the law enforcers admitted, but the location of the major press conference was yet to be determined. Shamel walked into the ER and immediately began looking around for Preacher as well as members of his unit.

"Excuse me ma'am, I'm searching for a Preacher Haynes." Shamel said to one of the clerks.

"Is he one of the injured cops that were brought in?" she asked.

"Yes!" Shamel replied enthusiastically.

"Sweetie, there's so many cops here, we don't even know which ones are the patients anymore! But head over to the trauma area, maybe you'll find him there. And by the way, thank you!" she replied.

"For?" Shamel asked puzzled.

"Helping to rid the city of those gun and drug dealers! We've got enough problems!"

That made Shamel feel real proud! He winked at the clerk and smiled, before heading towards the trauma area.

"Hey Sha!" Viper yelled out as Shamel was passing by one of the rooms.

"Viper! Man, you one of the last *brotha's* I thought would have gotten hurt!"

"I'm ok. Doctor said thanks to my big biceps, I suffered more tissue damage than muscle or bone! Still, I'm gonna be out for a while, so you're gonna have to *rock the bling* while I'm gone!"

At that moment, Sequoia walked into the room with Lavender.

"There you are! We didn't know what happened to you, Shamel. I saw your twin, and thought it was you that had gotten hurt!" Sequoia admonished.

"Yeah. It's bad enough this one caught a bullet!" Lavender sighed, rubbing Viper's un-injured arm.

"Do you know where Preacher is now?" Shamel eagerly asked.

"In the waiting room. I'll get him!" Sequoia said.

As soon as Sequoia walked out, the tour supervisor walked in slightly afterward.

"Great job everyone!" he boomed. Shamel, Lavender, and Viper replied with a unanimous **"Thank you!"**

"Listen. The Police Commissioner has decided to have the press conference back at One Police Plaza. They wanted to get a hold of the guns and drugs confiscated in the operation first to display them for the cameras. So as soon as you finish up here, hustle on down to 'Centre Street'.

"You got it." Shamel answered for everyone.

As the tour supervisor was leaving the room, Sequoia came back in with Preacher.

"Man, where have you been? I had everybody mistaking me for you! It felt good though!" Preacher said to Shamel, as the brothers hugged each other.

"Sorry bro. Had to run uptown!"

"I see! You done got all fresh and clean! Just leave the rest of us bloody and stinking, won't ya?" Preacher kidded.

"Hey, that was the tour supervisor, right? Sequoia asked Shamel.

"Yeah. He just wanted to tell us about the news conference."

"Be right back!" Sequoia hummed, as she ran off behind the tour supervisor.

Shamel just smiled, and began counting backwards.

"10, 9, 8, 7…"

Preacher gave Shamel a bewildered look, but just as Shamel got to number one, Sequoia re-entered the room with a dejected look on her face.

"Wouldn't give you any time off, right?" Shamel ribbed.

"You know, I really have to start getting hurt like you men!" Sequoia groaned.

"Look at it this way. The less time you spend out injured, the more criminals you can take off the streets!"

"And I suppose when it's you who's out, those same criminals are being good - just waiting for you to come back and get them!" Sequoia snapped.

"I didn't say all of that. But-"

"What Sha's trying to say is that the world is simply a better place with you in it." Preacher cut in.

"That's a load of crap, but I do like the way it sounds!" Sequoia replied.

"We better get going. Here's the key to the police cruiser, Sequoia. Viper, holla atcha later!" Shamel said.

Everyone gave their final good-byes before heading out. Sequoia and Lavender caught a ride from a marked unit back to the Brooklyn Marine terminal to retrieve the cruiser, while Preacher rode with Shamel in his car to downtown Manhattan, as they headed to One Police Plaza.

Chapter Thirty-eight

The press conference was about to begin. It was going to be broadcast live on the evening news. As reporters and camera persons jockeyed for good positions inside the conference room, technicians were providing sound checks of their microphones on the podium.

"Mic is live!"

"Mic is hot!"

"Give me a level." - And other broadcasting jargon could be heard as final preparations were being completed before they went on the air.

The Mayor, Police Commissioner, Commanding Officer of B.L.I.N.G., US Attorney General, Brooklyn district attorney, head of the Drug Enforcement Administration's New York division, Port Authority police chief, Rear Admiral Sum-Yam and Special Agent King as representatives of the U.S. Navy, Shamel and Preacher, and a last minute representative from the bureau of Alcohol, Tobacco, Firearms and Explosives all made up the body of interviewees for

'Operation Empty Clip' - which was now being referred to as 'Operation Clean State. (ATF and Explosives got offended that they weren't part of the process despite the time frame. Since it was more of a weapons haul than illicit drugs, DEA compromised and decided to give them credit too.) The name was also chosen for the effort to stop and rid the now disbanded M.A.D. Mafia Family's attempt to distribute drugs and guns throughout the East Coast, as that information was finally gleaned from Stefan himself, upon learning of Mstislav's demise. As soon as it hit 11pm, red lights on video cameras blinked on throughout the room. Various reporters from broadcast and cable news began speaking into their own mics and cameras. Radio and print media journalists were talking into digital and analog recorders. The press conference was underway.

"As Mayor of this great city, I can't begin to express the gratitude that I know is felt by everyone for 'Operation Clean State' having been such a success. But now I'm going to turn things over to the Police

Commissioner, who will give you all the specifics on the raid of the decade!"

The sound and brilliance of cameras flashing filled the room, as the mayor and police commissioner switched positions at the podium.

"Thank you, Mayor Applewitz. Good evening. Displayed on this table in front of you, is a small sample of all that was confiscated during the raid. This represents only a fraction of the drugs and weapons that were destined for the streets of Boston, and eventually New York again as well as other eastern municipalities. With the assistance of the Port Authority police, we also managed to nab additional members of this crime family who were coming over the George Washington Bridge with a supplemental shipment of firearms in an armored van. The estimated street value of this bust on the weapons alone is equivalent to a total of over $330 million!"

There was a loud gasp from the crowd, as reporters raised their hands to ask questions. The mayor signaled for quiet, as the police commissioner continued.

"To my knowledge, this crime family took in over 30 million annually. I speculate the extra 300 came from this unusually large shipment of the smuggling process by the military's involvement. Our operation was a combined effort of various agencies which participated in shutting down the violent *Mad Mafia*, headed by a now deceased Mstislav Afanasi Diviodich – did I get the name right, Agent King?" Agent King along with Shamel and Preacher murmured "Yes.", then he continued... "Who I understand was the mastermind of this corruption."

"Commissioner, was he military or civilian?" a reporter yelled out.

"To my understanding he was a civilian." the Commissioner replied.

"How did the military get involved?" another reporter yelled out.

"Well, for that I need to turn you over to representatives of the military. I'd like to introduce you to naval officer Rear Admiral Sum-Yam from the Pegasus carrier group, and Special agent King from Naval Criminal Investigative Service."

There was a low murmur from the crowd, as Tristian instead of Rear Admiral Sum-Yam actually came up to the podium next.

"Good evening. I'm Special Agent King, NCIS. We were initially tipped off to this crime family by a Seaman who was arrested in a drug bust at Little Creek Amphibious Base. That led to a full-scale investigation, which included frequent random drug searches. Our efforts paid off once we were introduced to Detective Haynes from the NYPD's special narcotics division, appropriately dubbed BLING..."

There was a small utterance of laughter from the crowd, as even Tristian chuckled, then continued.

"Excuse me. We met New York Detective Haynes <u>and</u> Detective Haynes from the Alexandria, Virginia PD narcotics unit. They're twin brothers by the way. Pretty cool. But thanks in part to both of these fine detectives, NCIS was able to apprehend the military associates of the *MAD* crime family, and bring them to justice."

"Agent King, who was responsible for the raid at the Brooklyn Marine terminal?" another reported yelled out.

"Once again, it was a combined endeavor from various agencies, but I'll turn the podium over to NYPD Detective Haynes now, who can give you more information on his unit which spearheaded the strike."

Again there was a murmur from the crowd, as Tristian and now Shamel switched positions.

"Thank you, Special Agent King. Good evening everyone. I'm Detective Shamel Haynes, NYPD-BLING division. We certainly can't take all the credit for shutting down the *MAD Mafia family*. Our efforts are concentrated here in New York. It was purely by chance that BLING was able to get involved and break up Mr. Diviodich's gang. If anything, I'll let you speak to my twin brother who's the real key in our successful takedown of the *MMF*."

As they switched positions, Preacher whispered to Shamel, "Why are you putting me up to this? I didn't do anything special!"

"Just get your 15 minutes of fame!" Shamel whispered back, as he continued shuffling to the side.

Preacher came up to the podium, adjusted the microphone, cleared his throat, and then began speaking.

"(Ahem), hello. I'm Detective Preacher Haynes, Alexandria, VA narcotics unit. Um, wow. I don't really know what to say. If it wasn't for certain events that occurred in DC, we probably wouldn't be standing here tonight. I was fortunate to participate in a raid on a drug den with the Washington, DC Metro police that subsequently led to the apprehension of an associate of the MMF, which finally resulted in the unification of our agencies to halt their crime spree. Call me modest or humble, but I was only doing my job."

All of the reporters tried to speak at once, but Preacher picked one female in particular out of the cluster and took her question.

"Detective, how do you justify condemning a man in the court of public opinion, when no trial has been held?"

That comment took the entire room by surprise, especially Preacher.

"I don't follow you." he replied to the reporter.

"At no point in time did you or anyone else state, 'these **alleged** members'. How can you be so sure that you've got the right people?" the reporter concluded.

That riled Preacher very much.

"Hey - you know what? Turn these damn cameras off! Listen here, lady," Preacher directed his discord towards the reporter in an unsympathetic tone of voice. "I've seen what drugs have done to entire communities! Including the tragedy at the elementary school and other schools across the nation, I've seen what gun violence has done to communities! I witnessed crack addicts trying to sell everything from obviously stolen goods to their own bodies to infants! I've seen babies in withdrawal, and probably seen even more go into unmarked graves! I made arrests of addicts who swore they were getting into a detox program, only to re-arrest them sometimes days later, making the same claim! I've been to funerals for neighborhood youth whose lives were claimed by gun violence! And finally, I have had to personally inform some mother on occasion, that her only child was caught in the crossfire of a shootout between rival drug gangs and gun runners, then stand there while she broke down crying and screaming, beating on me, asking 'Why?'! As much as the guns are an issue, this is an ***Anti-Drug Matter,*** something that you probably know nothing about, living in your own sheltered society! So when an antagonist such as yourself stands there boldface and questions whether I believe that I have the right people behind bars for 'dealing', the only thing I have to say is walk a mile in my damn shoes, and experience the blisters! As far **as I'm** concerned, this press conference is over!"

Preacher slapped the microphone back from his mouth, and stormed off. Even the Mayor was insulted. He stepped back up to the podium and sternly said

"No more questions!" before everyone left the platform.

Shamel hesitated for a moment, then ran after Preacher.

Chapter Thirty-nine

Preacher forcefully pushed the door open as he made his way outside. He brushed through a small throng of reporters who hadn't made it inside to the press conference, without saying a word. Shamel came outside almost on Preacher's heels. As he too brushed past the reporters, he ran and caught up to Preacher who was walking very briskly in silence. Shamel decided to just walk along with him in silence, until Preacher felt he was ready to speak. Preacher went to the crosswalk on Centre Street where the light was already green. Crossing over to the island, Preacher then began to make his way up to the Brooklyn Bridge. Only after arriving on the pedestrian walkway of the bridge did he finally stop. He noticed a small stone on the walkway and in a show of revulsion kicked it off into the river down below. Shamel figured now it was time to open his mouth…

"Man that was some display! For a minute, I thought you were me! You're supposed to be the laid-back one."

Preacher turned to Shamel and griped, "There may as well have been guns aimed at me, because that was the worst ambush I've ever experienced! What has the world come to, when we as law enforcers get persecuted for trying to maintain novus ordo seclorum? In every courtroom in America, the phrase 'In God We Trust' is displayed in plain sight for all to see once you enter. But God isn't the one being consulted when it comes down to the plea bargains and deal cutting!"

"I hate to be a killjoy, but we haven't been capable of maintaining law and order ever since Cain took Abel's life!" Shamel countered.

"You're missing my point, Sha! I don't know where that reporter came from with that asinine comment, but I feel much unappreciated for my efforts at trying to protect and serve! It goes back to what you said when we were interrogating Seryoga. All of these things in some way or another are responsible for our father's death!"

"Oh, you remember that!"

"Yes! That same night of the incident back when we were kids, dad and I had a talk. You were already in bed when I asked dad what he would have done if someone stuck a gun in his face. He said that as far as his job went, the official policy was to give up the money. They were only supposed to pull out their guns as a last resort in self-defense. I'm willing to bet both of our salaries, that at least one of those robbers had a drug habit."

To Shamel's surprise, Preacher suddenly became emotional. He clenched both of his fists, as tears welled up in his eyes and he continued speaking.

"Dad never came home again after that night, because justice failed! The system failed! Remember, the only surviving robber out of the entire group had an extensive rap sheet, which up until dad's killing, didn't include murder! Even though this guy's going to be incarcerated for the rest of his life, we had to grow up without the fulfillment of seeing our parents live a long life together! That bothers me, because it's not like they were divorced, or he just walked out of our lives, or died in an accident! He was stolen from us! That's something I personally cannot and will not ever forgive that bastard who killed him for!"

Preacher took his hand and brushed away at his eyes. He then walked over to the railing, and peered back at the city. Shamel walked over to Preacher, and threw his arm around him.

"You know Shamel? I know I live in Maryland now. Work in Virginia. But when I look at New York, I can't help but wonder if we are making a difference across the board. I think back to that day we ran into those older teen kids."

"Literally, right?" Shamel joked.

"Yeah, literally." Preacher continued. "Did it ever occur to you, that as narcotics cops, this is another form of saying 'no'? I think subconsciously, we both joined narcotics because we're still saying 'no'."

"True, but much like someone who works as a pharmacist, we have easy and constant access to drugs." Shamel said.

"But you also have a choice. The same way we could have chosen a life of crime, is the same way you can choose to do drugs. As much as we're around this stuff, do you find it hard to resist, or isn't the temptation non-existent?"

"I have no desire to partake of what we arrest other people for."

"Neither do I, which only proves my point. (Sigh) I can't help but wonder if all of our efforts as law enforcers combined aren't just helping to put food on our families' tables and pay our bills. I wonder if somewhere, somehow, a difference is actually being made."

"Trust me when I tell you, there is. You and I could have elected to work for transit. Or we could have gotten jobs with private firms, or even in education. But I know within my heart, that no matter how many 'Mstislav's' of the world we put away, there's always going to be another one waiting to take his place. This is where the difference is being made. Regardless of the number of 'Mstislavs' out here, there will always be a

Haynes ready to take them down. A fat cat in between two hungry dogs is nothing more than a 'happy meal' without the cholesterol!"

Preacher turned to Shamel and quipped, "Bro, you crazy!"

"Just as crazy as you! We're two brothers from the same mother!"

"Funny, I remember saying that somewhere!"

Preacher and Shamel laughed, then embraced each other in a hug.

"Man bro, I love you, and I'm glad you're my brother!" Preacher said to Shamel.

"Same goes for me. I'm glad you're my brother, and I love you man!"

They patted each other on the back, then Shamel said to Preacher, "Let's head back in and see if they formed a lynch mob for that reporter!"

"I'm with you. I didn't recognize her, but think her ID read 'The National Liar'."

"And you got mad at her? You should have known she was there to twist everything you say! The

National Liar only hires journalists who finish in the bottom percentile of their class, or have been fired from more prestigious publications!"

"So I overreacted and got mad for nothing, huh?"

"No. I overheard the mayor say he had to go take a *shit* anyway!"

Both preacher and Shamel laughed themselves silly, as they headed off the bridge back towards One Police Plaza.

Chapter Forty

The next day back at Floyd Bennett Field, Shamel was giving his final farewells to Preacher, Tristian, Zachary, and the rest of the NCIS team.

"Shamel, it was a pleasure working with you. On behalf of NCIS and the Navy, we're deeply indebted to you and your unit. Of course, we owe thanks to you as well, Preacher." Tristian extolled.

"It was a group effort. I'm sure BLING will be in close contact with NCIS as the stragglers and co-conspirators are rounded up." Shamel replied.

"I still say I didn't do anything out of the ordinary. Guess I'm a bit desensitized to grandeur." Preacher said.

"Well, there's always the 'what ifs'. What if you hadn't gone on that raid?" Tristian asked.

"What if we missed you at your precinct, since you were actually on vacation?" Zachary added.

"What if we hadn't made it to New York before they got that shipment of drugs and guns out of the city?" Preacher wondered.

"What if - Elvis, wasn't King?" Shamel taunted.

Preacher couldn't resist. He knew what was coming next, and joined Shamel, as they both said in unison, **"Uh thank-you! Thank-you very much!"**

Zachary made a face, but Tristian just smirked and replied, "Take care." before nudging Zachary to board. Preacher turned his attention back to Shamel and said, "Gotta be getting back. You know Claudine's *hot* with me. She's mad at you too. Even though she understands, all she kept saying when I was on the phone with her was, 'But you didn't have to go to New York. Every time you get with Shamel, ya get into trouble!' Then she told me to tell you to 'Hurry back, and make sure Nova's with you!' Crazy woman! But anyway, do you want me to send your things, UPS?"

"Ah, just hold them till the next time we come down. It's not like I'm hurting for clothes or anything! By the way, did you manage to speak with anyone from the DEA despite all this chaos?" Shamel replied.

"As a matter of fact, yes! The deputy director from the New York field office said he would contact HR back in Washington and inform them of my participation in this joint op. He told me that they liked seeing selfless acts of valor and teamwork, and this may just get me hired a little faster!" Preacher affirmed.

"Final boarding call for Preacher Haynes as this is the last flight out of Brooklyn today! Come on!" Tristian called out.

"I'd better go. Like I told you before, I love you bro." Preacher said to Shamel.

"And I love you, bro. Holla at me when you get home."

"No doubt. Peace."

"Preach! One more thing real quick."

Preacher looked at Shamel inquisitively.

"What do you call a pig that just got off a plane?"

"Jet slab?" Preacher asked.

"No. Try *swine flew*!" Shamel countered.

As the two brothers laughed, they engaged in one final cultural handshake/hug combination before Preacher boarded the jet. As the jet became airborne, Shamel waived and watched it until it was out of sight.

He then got into his car, and drove uptown to his precinct for debriefing on yesterday's occurrence.

Chapter Forty-one

It was the end of Shamel's tour. He had just completed some paperwork on an arrest he made earlier in the morning when Sequoia sauntered into the room.

"Go on home, Sha. I'll take this perp down to central booking." she insisted.

"You sure? It's my arrest. Besides, you're awfully enthused for a person willing to go where there are a lot of stinky cells!"

Sequoia coyly smiled, then said, "Don't know why you all up in 'rome' *bizness* but I confess. I didn't tell you earlier, but I have a new boyfriend."

"Really? So you **did** get rid of 'ol boy from Wall Street!" Shamel replied astounded.

"I told you I would! Anyway, we're meeting in 'the Village' for drinks, so I figured since you live uptown; you wouldn't have to go out of your way."

"It's no bother, but thanks. So where did you meet this guy?"

Sequoia giggled and bowed her head in humility. She then looked up at Shamel and said, "Would you believe at the raid?"

"Oh no you didn't!" Shamel guffawed.

"Yeah, I did! He's a merchant Marine. He saw me coming out of the terminal with that suspect and said to me, 'I like the way you handle your men!' Of course we couldn't actually talk at that moment, so we just quickly exchanged numbers and agreed to call one another once we had time."

"Only you could meet someone at a raid!" Shamel teased.

Sequoia folded her arms and replied, "It's no different than a guy meeting a woman at a funeral."

"I wouldn't know! I don't do things like that." Shamel countered.

"Come on Sha, be happy for me!" Sequoia implored.

"I am! I'm just wondering now if he's going to be the one to christen those sheets!" Shamel joked.

Sequoia bent down, and seductively whispered into Shamel's ear, "Wouldn't you like to know?" before quickly flicking her tongue in it.

"Aiight! Keep it up; you won't be making it to 'the Village!" Shamel playfully admonished.

"I'm going! I'm going! Take care, Shamel. See you tomorrow. I'll let you know how my date went."

"Please do. Be careful, have fun, and make sure *Captain Morgan* doesn't deliberately 'spice' <u>your</u> rum!"

"See? You don't even know his name, and already you're criticizing."

"Just protect your drinks."

"You don't know his - name…" Sequoia replied in song.

"GHB isn't that hard to obtain."

"You don't know his - name…" Sequoia sang again, as she walked away.

"Hey Sequoia! What's his name anyway?" Shamel yelled after her, but Sequoia just kept walking and repeated one more time,

"You don't know his - name..." before fading from view.

Shamel laughed to himself, closed up his desk, and signed out for the night. On his way home, Preacher happened to call him on his cell phone...

"Hey bro! What's cracking?" Shamel asked upon answering.

"(Chuckle) Seems like you've been!"

"Ok, what are you talking about?" Shamel said.

"All I'm going to say, is you need to get home as soon as you can. Nova called Claudine, and Claudine called me screaming all in my ear! I'm still having trouble hearing!"

"I'm guessing it's nothing serious, considering Nova didn't call me." Shamel said, with a bit of vagueness.

"Well Sha, all on going to say is, try to act surprised. Normally you would have found out first, but I guess Nova was just so excited she couldn't contain herself. Gotta go, but we'll talk again soon - big daddy!"

"Shamel pulled the phone back from his ear and glanced at it befuddled, as Preacher hung up. He shrugged his shoulders and pondered if it was a new job Nova found that Preacher was hinting at. As Shamel pulled onto his block, he was fortunate once again to be able to park right in front of his building. After locking up the car, he headed upstairs to the apartment and opened the door, calling out Nova's name as he entered.

"Nova?"

"In the bathroom!" Nova yelled back.

Shamel went to the bathroom, and saw Nova bent over the sink. She looked flushed, but displayed a wide smile upon seeing Shamel.

"Hey babycakes, are you all right?" Shamel asked, very concerned.

"Yes! I've been *throwing up* though. Thought it was something I ate, but then I remembered I didn't get my thirty-day 'red alert'. So I took an EPT." Nova then stood up, and handed Shamel the indicator. "Hope you like symbols, or should I say the symbol?" Nova asked keenly.

Shamel took it from her, and looked at the window. It displayed a blue 'plus' sign.

"You're pregnant! YOU'RE PREGNANT!" Shamel yelled excitedly, as Nova rapidly nodded her head up and down with a big smile. Shamel couldn't contain his exhilaration. He grabbed Nova up in a big hug, carried her out of the bathroom and spun her around. "Nova, that's great! I'm honored to be your baby's daddy!"

"Me too!" Nova replied. Then suddenly, Nova became very melancholic. "Oh Sha, I'm sorry. Really it's a bad time. With me still not working, and you want to buy a house and-"

Shamel cut Nova off in her sentence. "Nova, nova, nova! Listen to me. First of all, I love you, and you know I got your back. Second, if we sit here and contemplate when it's going to be the right time to have a child, the time will never be right. I'm not about to let you feel guilty or sorry for this blessing. In fact, I feel guilty because I'd rather do this the right way. But since no one is promised tomorrow, I want you to make that conversion I mentioned, today!" Upon that, Shamel got down on one knee, looked up into Nova's beautiful mesmerizing hazel eyes and proclaimed, "Nova Springfield, will you accept my last name as you own, with or without a hyphen?"

Nova could have fainted… "YES!" she hollered at the top of her lungs, and tightly hugged Shamel as he rose up to embrace her as well. Tears of joy streamed down her face, as she and Shamel continued to hold each other close. They engaged in a passionate kiss, then Shamel turned Nova around and embraced her in his arms while nuzzling her neck.

Nova decided that now was the time to put her bid in…

"Shamel?"

"Mmm, yes, babycakes?"

"When you do get my ring, can I have three carats?"

"THREE!"

Shamel released his hold of Nova and jumped back. Nova turned around just in time to see the look of astonishment on Shamel's face. She then said to him in a reassuring tone of voice,

"I'm worth it!"

"I know you are, Nova. You really are. But damn! Three?"

Nova smiled and turned around, snuggling back into Shamel's arms.

"Well can I at least get two and one-quarter?"

Shamel groaned.

"Don't groan at me!" Nova begged.

Shamel just groaned again.

"Two?"

"Ok, two." Shamel joyfully sighed, as he relented.

"Two and a half?" Nova pushed.

"ONE." Shamel adamantly declared.

"Ok, ok, ok! I'll take the two!" - Nova giggled. She then cooed softly, "Do you know my ring size?"

"No." Shamel replied. "But if it's the same size as your feet, I'll figure it out after measuring them with my tongue!" he said, kissing her neck.

"You nasty!" Nova purred.

"Well why don't we take a shower together? Like I always say, 'a clean body – is the sign of a dirty lover!'"

Nova and Shamel embraced in in a kiss, as they both tottered back into the bathroom. Minutes later, with their clothes off and the water running, amid the rising steam inside the shower…

People as far south back in Brooklyn could swear they heard a woman screaming – in total and pure ecstasy.

*****

www.ingramcontent.com/pod-product-compliance
Lightning Source LLC
LaVergne TN
LVHW010555100826
845148LV00014B/2720

* 9 7 8 0 6 1 5 7 8 2 5 5 3 *